Safe Food for You and Your Family

written for
The American Dietetic Association

by
Mildred M. Cody, Ph.D., R.D.

**CHRONIMED
PUBLISHING**

Library of Congress Cataloging-in-Publication Data

Safe food for you and your family / The American Dietetic Association

     p.   cm.

Includes index.

ISBN 0-471-34699-3 $5.95

Edited by: Jeff Braun
Cover Design: Terry Dugan Design
Text Design & Production: David Enyeart
Art/Production Manager: Claire Lewis

Published by
Chronimed Publishing
P.O. Box 59032
Minneapolis, MN 55459-9686

Mildred M. Cody, Ph.D., R.D.
Georgia State University
Atlanta, Georgia

The American Dietetic Association

Reviewers:
Lorri Fishman, M.S., R.D.
National Center for Nutrition and Dietetics
Chicago, Illinois

Pat Kendall, Ph.D., R.D.
Colorado State University
Fort Collins, Colorado

April C. Mason, Ph.D.
Purdue University
West Lafayette, Indiana

Technical Editor:

Betsy Hornick, M.S., R.D.
The American Dietetic Association
Chicago, Illinois

Safe Food for You and Your Family

The American Dietetic Association is the largest group of food and nutrition professionals in the world. As the advocate of the profession, the ADA serves the public by promoting optimal nutrition, health, and well-being.

For expert answers to your nutrition questions, call the ADA/National Center for Nutrition and Dietetics Hot Line at (800) 366 1655, and speak directly with a registered dietitian (RD), listen to recorded messages, or obtain a referral to an RD in your area.

NOTICE:

CONSULT A HEALTH CARE PROFESSIONAL

Readers are advised to seek the guidance of a licensed physician or health care professional before making changes in health care regimens, since each individual case or need may vary. This book is intended for informational purposes only and is not for use as an alternative to appropriate medical care. While every effort has been made to ensure that the information is the most current available, new research findings, being released with increasing frequency, may invalidate some data.

Contents

Introduction   **1**

Chapter 1—The Basics   **5**

Are You at Risk?
Causes of Foodborne Illness
How Does Food Become Contaminated?
The Time and Temperature Connection
Potentially Unsafe Foods
Mission Possible:
    Destroy the Disease-Causing Agents

Chapter 2—At Home   **25**

Selecting Food
Taking Food Home
Storing Foods at Home
Keeping the Kitchen Clean and Safe
Preparing Foods
Cooking Foods
Serving Foods
Leftovers
Handling Raw Meat and Poultry

Chapter 3—Away From Home   69
Packing Meals From Home
Picnics
Barbecues
Camping and Backpacking
Bringing Home the Catch
Holiday and Company Meals
Food Functions for Club, Community,
    and Religious Groups
Food Gifts
Childcare Centers

Chapter 4—Our Food Supply
is (Still) Changing   101
Food Additives
Pesticides
New Food Processes
Biotechnology

Chapter 5—Help! A Resource Guide   115

Appendix 1—Safety Recommendations for
Selected Foods   121

Appendix 2—Characteristics of Selected
Contaminants   139

Index   147

Introduction

Think back to the last time you experienced muscle aches, diarrhea, dizziness, or vomiting. Was it the flu? Or could it have been something you ate?

There's a good chance that your symptoms were caused by foodborne illness. Sometimes called food poisoning, foodborne illness results from eating contaminated food.

Contaminated food. The words alone make your stomach turn. They also spark thoughts of recent headlines about undercooked fast-food hamburgers, contaminated eggs, and unsanitary practices in food processing plants.

Fortunately, these incidences are quite rare. America has one of the world's safest food supplies. At each step in the food chain—from farm to food manufacturer to market—strict regulations are in place to ensure safe food for

1

consumers. But when the system breaks down and foodborne illness strikes a large number of people, it makes the news.

What you rarely if ever see on the front page are stories about foodborne illness that strike individual households. Apparently, a few people affected at one time is not very newsworthy. On top of this, most of these incidents go unreported.

That doesn't mean foodborne illness at home is any less serious. In fact, it is much more common than large outbreaks. Foodborne illness in general is probably more common than you think. Each year about one in every ten Americans has an illness caused by food. Most of these cases result in simple stomachaches or diarrhea. Some are more serious. About 9,000 cases result in death each year. Some also result in long term problems, such as birth defects, arthritis, hemolytic uremic syndrome, and Guillain-Barre syndrome.

A Preventable Problem

Fortunately, you can do a lot to protect yourself and your family from foodborne illnesses—especially at home.

Food safety requires more than a heavy dose of common sense. With so many foods and so many possible situations, food safety depends on specific information and guidelines for specific situations. And that's what you'll get in *Safe Food for You and Your Family.*

Chapter 1 starts by covering the all-important basics of food safety, such as how contamination occurs, how to destroy contaminants, and the "7 Commandments of Food Safety."

From there, **Chapter 2** moves into the specifics of food safety, including: how to spot the safest foods at the supermarket, how to store them, and then how to prepare, cook, and serve safe foods at home, even leftovers.

In **Chapter 3,** you'll learn about eating and serving safe foods away from home, whether for a picnic, camp outing, community function, or at a childcare center.

The effects of food additives, irradiation, and other new food preparation processes are covered in **Chapter 4,** including the latest information on foods created from biotechnology.

Finally, in **Appendix 1** you will find a concise listing of the specific cooking, storage, and other safety recommendations for selected foods. To further help you guard against contaminants, **Appendix 2** summarizes the characteristics of common food contaminants, including what symptoms they might produce.

As you'll discover, safe food precautions go beyond the kitchen. They apply everywhere food is grown, sold, prepared, and stored. With *Safe Food for You and Your Family*, you can make sure you and your family are safe every step of the way.

Chapter 1

The Basics

Food safety has come a long way, especially in recent years. Not only do scientists know more about potential dangers, but we as consumers are also more aware of food safety issues. *Salmonella* and *E. coli 0157:H7* have practically become household words.

Still, there's a lot of misinformation out there. Some people mistakenly think it's up to the government alone to assure a safe food supply. True, the United States Department of Agriculture and other agencies set food safety regulations and provide training and educational materials on food safety. They also monitor industries that produce and market foods. In a typical inspection, the inspector looks for evidence that regulations are followed. One weakness in this system is that these inspections are sporadic and may not catch all potential problems.

Regardless, once you buy foods from a grocery store, restaurant, or other retailer, food safety becomes your responsibility. In other words, it's up to you to select, store, prepare, and serve safe foods for you and your family.

Are You at Risk?

Everyone is susceptible to foodborne illness—some more than others, though. People most susceptible are those with an impaired immune system or serious health problems. Besides being more susceptible, foodborne illness also can have a more severe impact on these people. Individuals at greatest risk for foodborne illness include:

- persons with HIV and AIDS
- persons with cancer, especially those undergoing drug or radiation treatments
- persons with liver, diabetes, chronic kidney, inflammatory bowel, or stomach diseases
- persons who are taking steroid medication
- pregnant women
- infants and children
- elderly

If you are at greater risk of foodborne illness, be extra careful with food and talk with your doctor or a registered dietitian about any special precautions you should take. Besides your health status, other factors also contribute to the incidence of foodborne illness:

Our food supply is changing. The desire for convenient foods continues to grow. We're eating more and more foods prepared from a variety of sources. Many new foods are available in the marketplace—as partially prepared, or precooked ready-to-serve, or speed scratch, where you finish the preparation by adding one or two ingredients. Because these newer foods look like familiar preserved foods or home-cooked foods, it may not be obvious that they require special care. Reading labels for handling instructions is essential!

New food packaging techniques allow retailers to offer prepared foods that can be refrigerated longer than we've been used to. This is made possible by vacuum packaging or modified atmosphere packaging where oxygen in the package is replaced with carbon dioxide or nitrogen. These techniques slow spoilage, discoloration, and the growth of many bacteria. This new packaging is used for fully

7

cooked roast chicken, "fresh" pastas, sauces and many other foods.

Foods may be processed four to six weeks before the "sell by" or "use by" date. These dates assume that the product is refrigerated properly throughout its shelf life. Also many of these foods do not require additional cooking or thorough heating before consumption.

To use refrigerated, prepared foods safely:
- When purchasing, make sure that the food is cold and the packaging is intact. Never buy refrigerated, prepared foods that have torn packages or that have been repackaged.
- Purchase these foods last, and take them home quickly. Refrigerate them as soon as you get home.
- Purchase foods by their "sell by" date. Use foods by their "use by" date. *(For more on product dating, see page 38.)*
- Read the label and follow storage and cooking or heating instructions carefully.
- If you freeze these products, do so as soon as possible after purchase.

Food safety education is limited. Fewer food preparation skills are being taught in school and at

8

home. This means that tomorrow's foodservice workers are likely to have very little food preparation skills or food safety knowledge. They may mishandle foods without knowing it. Even your own family members may not have "common sense" about food safety. Although most foodborne disease is preventable, you must know what to do in order to prevent it!

New disease-causing microorganisms continue to emerge. Our grandparents did not worry about *Listeria monocytogenes, Campylobacter jejuni, Salmonella enteritidis* or *Escherichia coli 0157:H7.* But these disease-causing microorganisms carried in food have made it onto the public health "least wanted" list. They are the organisms that our national health objectives have targeted.

Causes of Foodborne Illness
Foodborne illness can be caused by:

Toxic chemicals naturally present in food.
Although foods contain toxic substances, we have learned to recognize, avoid, or treat those foods. For example, rhubarb leaves are very toxic, so we eat only the stems. And

9

naturally-occurring toxins are found in certain seafoods and mushrooms.

Toxic chemicals in the environment.
Environmental contaminants entering food and causing foodborne illness is sporadic. For example, fish may become contaminated by mercury and other industrial chemical waste. To reduce this risk, follow all advisories that accompany sportfishing licenses, and never eat the internal organs of fish. And always buy food from reliable sources.

Pesticide residues and food additives. Food additives and pesticides are tested for safety before they can be approved for food use. Safety of all pesticides and food additives is regulated by federal, state and local governments. Ongoing studies of these chemicals continue even after their approval. They can be removed from use if they become problems. *(Also see page 104.)*

Although general use is safe, some additives are harmful to certain people. For example, aspartame should be avoided by individuals with the disease phenylketonuria (PKU), and high levels of sulfites should be avoided by people with asthma.

Ingredient labels contain information if you're trying to avoid a certain additive. *(Also see page 102.)*

Pathogenic (disease-causing) microorganisms.
By far, the most common cause of foodborne illness in the United States is disease-causing microorganisms, which include bacteria, viruses, parasites and molds. Bacteria cause over 90 percent of all cases and over 90 percent of the deaths from foodborne illness. *Appendix 2 provides detailed information on certain bacteria and other pathogens and how to reduce your risk of illness from them.*

To cause foodborne illness in a healthy person, disease-causing microorganisms or chemicals must be present in food at levels capable of causing illness. This amount is different for different chemicals and microorganisms. For example, it takes only a few cells of *E. coli* bacteria to cause illness, but it typically takes thousands of salmonella. It is also different for different people. A small amount of salmonellae can cause foodborne illness in the very young, the elderly, pregnant women or immune-suppressed individuals, but may not cause any problems for a healthy adult.

Four major factors determine the reaction to a contaminated food:

- the type of bacteria or toxin,
- how extensively the food was contaminated,
- how much food was eaten, and
- the person's susceptibility.

How Does Food Become Contaminated?

Bacteria, viruses, parasites, or toxic chemicals can contaminate (become a part of) foods during production, transport, preparation, or service. Sometimes contamination is a natural part of producing foods, but often times it can be avoided.

Keep in mind that bacteria are present everywhere around us—on our skin, in the soil, in animals—so it's perfectly normal for bacteria to be present in some foods. When food that contains bacteria is mishandled, however, problems can occur.

Bacteria and other pathogens or chemicals can also become part of foods at various points.

During production. During growth, plants are exposed to naturally occurring soil- and water-borne pathogens from sewage, raw manure, and pesticides. Also, many plants contain naturally-occurring chemicals that are toxic. Food animals carry disease-causing bacteria normally (just as we do). Therefore, meats can be contaminated during slaughter and may have parasites in their tissues. Milk can also become contaminated during milking.

From other foods or utensils, surfaces, and equipment. Foods can become contaminated by contact with unclean objects or raw foods. This is called cross contamination because inanimate objects must "cross paths" or touch each other for it to occur. Cross contamination contributes to foodborne disease in almost half of bacterial outbreaks. Common examples of cross contamination include:
- using the same knife and/or cutting surface to prepare raw and cooked foods,
- using a contaminated sink for thawing meat or cleaning salad greens, or
- using uncooked meat marinade as a sauce.

By food handlers. People may contaminate unprotected food by touching it or by sneezing or coughing on it. Washing hands thoroughly is the first defense against bacteria and other toxic agents.

By pests and pets. Pests and pets can bring bacteria, viruses, and parasites from garbage, dirt, or sewage into kitchens or picnic areas. It is best to keep even healthy pets away from food preparation and service areas. To reduce contamination by pests, keep everything neat and clean because bugs like to live and lay their eggs in small areas. Since they require very little food and hide easily, it is difficult to eliminate pests once they have infested an area. You may choose to call a licensed exterminator. If you choose to exterminate the pests yourself, be sure to follow all safety precautions listed on the product, especially around food and food storage and preparation areas.

The Time and Temperature Connection

For most chemicals and some pathogens, the levels that originally occur in foods do not increase over time. However, bacteria can multiply to dangerous numbers. To survive and multiply, bacteria need time and the right conditions: food, moisture, and a temperature that promotes growth. Many need oxygen, too. Since most foodborne illnesses are caused by bacteria, their growth must be controlled to reduce risk of disease.

Temperature. The "danger zone" is the temperature range that bacteria grow the fastest. This range is from 40°F to 140°F. At temperatures below 40°F (refrigerator and freezer temperatures) bacteria grow slowly, if at all. At temperatures between 140°F and 160°F bacteria grow very slowly, and at temperatures above 160°F bacteria are destroyed. In general though, if food feels comfortable to the touch, it is probably in the danger zone. Most food serving and storage recommendations are based on keeping foods out of the danger zone. It is best to use a food thermometer to measure the temperature of foods during cooking and before serving.

Time. Under the right conditions, bacteria double in number every 20 to 30 minutes. The longer food is allowed to remain in the danger zone, the more disease-causing microorganisms will be present in the food. Generally, 2 hours is the maximum amount of time that a cooked food or raw food of animal origin should remain in the danger zone temperature.

Potentially Unsafe Foods

Almost all foods have the potential to cause disease if contaminated or not handled properly. However, it is unlikely that everyone who tastes or eats a contaminated food will become ill. First, you may not consume enough bacteria or disease-causing agent to you make you sick. Second, healthy bodies can often fight back.

Bacteria and molds can grow on susceptible foods, while parasites and viruses can be a part of food, but do not increase in numbers in food. Remember, the right conditions (time, temperature, moisture, nutrients, and oxygen) are needed for most bacteria to survive and multiply. Conditions that help to slow the growth of most bacteria include salt, sugar, acid, and lack of oxygen.

Foods of animal origin—raw meat, poultry, fish, eggs, and raw (unpasteurized) milk—are the most common food sources of bacteria. But foods in other food groups can also be potentially unsafe—that is, they can support the growth of bacteria, if mishandled. *Appendix 1 contains specific tips for storage and preparation of food to prevent growth of bacteria and molds.*

Meat-fish-poultry-dried bean-egg-nuts group. This group of foods has the nutrients that can support rapid growth of bacteria. Dried beans are not potentially hazardous until they are rehydrated. Properly dried nuts and nut butters are not a problem, but a moldy product can be. Eggs and other animal products—raw, cooked, or pasteurized—can support bacterial growth if they're not handled properly. Once canned meats, fish, and poultry are opened, proper handling is especially important.

Milk-cheese-yogurt group. These foods also have the nutrients required for bacteria and mold to grow. Some milk products, such as yogurt and cultured buttermilk, have enough acid to reduce bacteria and mold growth, but they can still be potentially unsafe.

Breads, cereals, and grains group. Within this group, certain foods have the nutrients to support rapid growth of bacteria and molds. They

17

do not have any acid to slow bacterial growth. The form of the food determines whether or not it is potentially unsafe. In their dried forms grains, flours, and pastas do not support bacterial growth. Once rehydrated and cooked, they can. For example, dried rice is safe, but cooked rice is potentially unsafe. Newer refrigerated pastas can support bacterial growth because they are not dried.

Fruit group. Fruits do not contain all of the nutrients required for bacteria to grow, and they

Does Spoiled Food Mean Unsafe Food?

When foods spoil, they taste, smell, or look different. Examples of food spoilage are soured milk, rancid butter, separated mayonnaise, even crushed potato chips. Spoiled foods will not necessarily cause foodborne illness. Spoilage warns us that food has been mistreated, possibly making it unsafe to eat. However, not all unsafe food is spoiled. Most food that causes foodborne illness looks and tastes good; otherwise, people would not eat it. If in doubt, though, it's safest to throw it out! Never taste a food that you suspect may be "bad."

usually contain enough acid to slow the growth. But, fresh fruits can have pathogens on their surfaces from dirt and handling; so washing fruits before eating is important. Moldy fruits and fruit products may contain disease-causing bacteria and molds and should be discarded.

Vegetable group. Vegetables also contain the nutrients that bacteria and molds need to grow. But, these nutrients are not usually available to bacteria and molds until vegetable cells are broken by bruising, mold growth, or cooking. That's why raw vegetables are not potentially hazardous, but cooked vegetables are. Dried vegetables—dried beans, corn, etc.—are not potentially unsafe until they are rehydrated. Once commercially canned vegetables are opened, proper handling is especially important. Frozen vegetables can support bacterial growth once they have thawed because they have been lightly pre-cooked.

Fats-sweets-alcohol group. Most foods that are largely fat, sugar, alcohol, or water do not support bacteria or mold growth. However, oils flavored with raw garlic, ginger, or herbs can support production of botulin toxin if a chemical preservative, added by a commercial manufacturer, is not present. That's why it's not a good idea to make your own flavored oil unless you plan to use it immediately. Commercial mayonnaise, an oil-based food made with pasteurized ingredients, has too much acid to encourage bacterial growth. However, homemade mayonnaise is potentially unsafe.

Home-canned foods. To be safe, home-canned foods must be carefully processed following guidelines similar to those for commercial processing and canning. Contact your local USDA Cooperative Extension Service for more information. Because many people do not follow appropriate procedures and regulators cannot verify that appropriate processes have been used, food prepared in a private home cannot be used or offered for human consumption in restaurants, grocery stores, or other public markets.

Mission Possible: Destroy the Disease-Causing Agents

Cooking, canning, and pasteurization kill bacteria, parasites, molds, and viruses. Cooking recommendations are designed to destroy these agents by bringing foods out of the danger zone and into the "kill range." Food processing methods—canning and pasteurization—also use heat to destroy bacteria, parasites, molds, and viruses. You cannot see, smell or taste disease-causing microorganisms, so use good quality thermometers to measure internal temperatures to check doneness in cooked meats, poultry, and casseroles.

Taking the guesswork out. Temperature is the best indicator of doneness for food. Temperature is the only measure of coldness for refrigerators and freezers. Temperature is one condition that determines whether bacteria can multiply and make you sick.

Using a thermometer correctly is the only way to reliably measure temperature. Thermometers for refrigerators and freezers may be mercury-in-glass, which are very fragile and not intended for measuring food temperatures. Types of thermometers for measuring food temperatures include:

- an oven-proof type,
- an instant-read or digital type used to give a quick reading when inserted into food,

21

- a pop-up type commonly found in poultry, or
- microwave-safe types designed for use in microwave ovens.

To use a thermometer for poultry insert it through the thickest part of the thigh muscle without touching the bone. The inner thigh is the area that heats most slowly. For turkey parts, insert the thermometer in the thickest area. For stuffed turkey, insert the thermometer into the center of the stuffing.

To use a thermometer for beef or other meats, insert it through the thickest part of the meat without touching the bone or allowing the thermometer to rest in fat.

To use a thermometer for casseroles, insert it in the thickest portion of the product.

To measure the temperature of microwaved foods, take the temperature in three or more places.

Note: When using an "instant read" thermometer, leave it in place several minutes for an accurate reading.

The 7 Commandments of Food Safety. With information and practice, you can make wise food safety decisions. Even for those foods of greatest concern, proper cooking can destroy the bacteria that may be present. Proper handling can reduce contamination of food and growth of disease-causing bacteria. In your own kitchen, you have more control of the safety of foods you cook. For foods that you eat without cooking, handling becomes more important, and you rely on the food industry and food inspection systems to keep food safe.

Be a knowledgeable consumer and follow the USDA's "7 Commandments of Food Safety" consistently.

1. Wash your hands before handling food.

2. Keep it safe, refrigerate.

3. Don't thaw food on the kitchen counter.

4. Wash hands, utensils, and surfaces again after coming in contact with raw meat, poultry, and fish.

5. Never leave perishable food out over 2 hours.

23

6. Thoroughly cook raw meat, poultry, and fish.

7. Freeze or refrigerate leftovers completely.

Chapter 2

At Home

As we mentioned earlier, home cooking causes millions of cases of foodborne illnesses across the country. So, what can you do to protect your family?

Selecting Food

Make safe food decisions. For starters, shop at reliable stores and markets, which are easier to regulate than temporary sites. Permanent facilities also are more likely to be pest-controlled and have employees who are trained to handle food. In other words, stay clear of people selling shellfish or other highly perishable foods from temporary roadside stands or the back of a truck. Always buy foods in good condition, such as fruit without cuts or bruises, cans without dents, and rock-solid ice cream. Inspect the groceries before you buy.

25

Look for:

Safe temperatures. Buy frozen food that is frozen solid. Packages of frozen corn, peas and other items should be separated; if they are in a solid block, they may have thawed and then refrozen. If there is "frost" inside the package, the foods may have been thawed and then refrozen. Packages that have lost their shape indicate damage, too. Refrigerated food should be very cold to the touch.

Should I Buy It?

Q *Is kosher food safer?*

A Kosher poultry and meats are salted during processing. This may eliminate some bacteria, but the flesh can still support growth of bacteria. Also, handling during marketing can recontaminate these products. Keep all fresh meats and poultry refrigerated or frozen until preparation and cook thoroughly.

Q *I saw some home-canned food for sale at a church bazaar. I thought it was illegal to sell*

Safe storage. All potentially hazardous foods should be refrigerated or frozen. An obvious example are canned hams that say "Keep refrigerated;" they should not be displayed in aisles. Eggs should be refrigerated. Foods should not be stored directly on the floor (except possibly cases of canned foods).

Safe packaging. Never buy food from a bulging or rusty can, a can with a damaged seal, or a tampered package. If you spot any on the shelves or when you get home, return them to the store manager.

home-canned food. The green beans looked good. Should I buy them?
A The government recommends that home-canned food not be sold. Most state and local codes also prohibit their sale. Church and social events are seldom monitored by inspectors because they are short, one-time happenings. It's also hard to monitor flea markets. It's risky to buy home-canned foods because you have no assurance that they were canned correctly.

27

Food protection. Many grocery stores and restaurants offer a variety of hot and cold foods buffet style or on a salad bar. These foods should be protected by sneeze guards or other covers. The areas around them should be clean, too.

Safe handling practices. You'd have to do some investigative work to verify this is being done, but grocery store workers should be washing their hands between tasks. This is particularly important in fresh bakery, meat, seafood, and deli departments, where workers may handle ready-to-eat foods that may not be cooked at home. When handling these foods, workers

Should I buy It?

Q *I found a frozen dinner on the shelf next to the canned soup at my grocery store. It was wet, but it seemed hard. It was the kind I was going to buy. Is it safe?*

A Only buy frozen foods from the freezer section. The package was "sweating" because it is much colder than the air surrounding it. If it is still very solid, it was probably just left there and is safe. Generally, it is best not to buy misplaced foods.

should have clean hands and wear disposable gloves. These gloves should be changed if they are damaged or when handlers begin a new task.

Clean facilities. If you see insects or rodents, there are probably many more. Insects are evidence of spilled food or opened containers. Droppings and chewed packages are a sure sign of rodents. By all means, alert the store manager if you see these pests or signs they are present.

Q *My neighbor's son has found a mushroom patch in the woods behind our house. I bought some from him, but they don't look like the kind from the store. Are they safe?*
A Eating wild mushrooms can be risky business. Many edible and poisonous species are hard to tell apart. Also, depending on the amount of toxin in the wild mushroom and the amount of mushrooms you eat, it could be toxic and even result in death.

29

When you are buying cooked, ready-to-eat or "take-out" food, watch for all of the above. Also, consider:

Keep hot foods hot and cold foods cold. Cooked food should not be allowed to remain at room temperature for longer than 2 hours. Leftovers from a restaurant meal may push this time, if you consider time in the kitchen and time to drive home. You increase your risk of foodborne illness if foods are kept at room temperature for longer than 2 hours.

Handling. If you use your hands or utensils that have been in your mouth to handle food, it should not be "saved" for a later meal. The bacteria that contaminate the food will grow quickly. And quick warming will not destroy bacteria or their toxins.

Cross-contamination. Cooked foods should not touch raw foods because raw foods have bacteria on their surfaces. For example, raw fish should not touch cooked shrimp. The fish will be cooked to destroy pathogens, but the shrimp will probably be eaten without further cooking. For this reason, cooked shrimp are displayed separately from the raw fish or other raw seafood.

Food packaging. Packaging protects food from becoming contaminated and from damage during marketing. Packaging also protects one food from contaminating another. Additionally, putting fresh meat, poultry, and seafood in plastic bags as overwrap will protect the other foods in your cart from drip. Intact packaging in the marketplace is essential for food safety. Take any food with damaged or tampered packaging to the store manager, such as

• bulging, seam-damaged, or rusty cans;
• foods in torn packaging that exposes the food; or
• foods that have been removed from original packaging or repackaged inappropriately. For example, a meat market may overwrap a leaking package. However, re-packaging a leaky ice cream carton is not appropriate because the ice cream should not have thawed.

Dates on foods. Generally, the dates on food apply only to unopened packages. Once a package is opened, it should be used in a reasonable time, depending on the food. *Appendix 1 provides information on using opened packages of food.*

Taking Food Home

Buy cold food last, get it home fast, and keep everything clean. When you're taking foods home, follow a few general rules:

Should I Buy It?

Q *I've seen people selling food from pushcarts in the park near my office. Is that food safe?*

A These street vendors should be licensed, just as restaurants are licensed. You are the last inspector. What you see and smell are important. It's easy to tell if ice cream and other frozen desserts are stored correctly; they should be firm with no evidence of melting. Look for steam coming from hot dogs held in water. Buns and condiments should be protected from fingers, flies, and sneezes. Packaged foods should be very cold or very hot. The vendor should not touch the food with bare hands because it is not likely that he or she cannot wash their hands effectively. Likewise,

Bag your food carefully at the grocery store check-out. If someone else bags your food for you, tell them how you want your foods separated and bagged. Put all frozen foods in the same bag to help keep them colder longer. Pack hot foods separately from cold foods. Put all the meat, poultry, and seafood together to help keep them from dripping on other foods. Avoid crushing foods or tearing their packag-

it may be difficult for you to wash fresh fruit; try fruit that can be peeled, such as a banana or a tangerine. Do not accept food that is out of date.

Q *I will be vacationing in South America this summer. Everyone has told me not to buy the "street food" but that I can still buy soft drinks from street vendors. Are the soft drinks safe?*
A Sanitation standards are different in different areas. Internationally-branded soft drinks are made with safe water. Remember to think of ice as a food, too. If you want your soft drink cold, buy it chilled; don't pour it over ice. (People who come to the United States often get sick from drinking water, too. We develop tolerances to different "bugs".)

ing. Don't bag cleaning aids or pest sprays with food.

Use a cooler to pack cold foods. If you travel longer than one hour to shop for food or if it takes you longer than thirty minutes to get home and the outside temperature is above 85°F, packing food in a cooler is a good idea. Use crushed ice or frozen blue ice packs to keep the temperature in the ice chest low. If you use crushed ice, use about one quarter as much ice as you have food, and surround the food completely. Package your foods in plastic bags before putting them on the ice. Place meats, poultry, and seafood at the bottom of the cooler to prevent them from dripping on other foods.

Keep foods clean. What have you carried in your car recently? If the answer is pets, recycling materials, or chemicals (fertilizers, pesticides, etc.), clean your car thoroughly before you go to the store. Do not allow foods to touch dirty car or truck storage or seat areas.

Keep refrigerated and frozen foods cold. The hottest part of the car is the trunk during the summer. Try to put your food in the passenger area instead or use a cooler.

Shop efficiently. Shop for refrigerated and frozen foods last so they have a better chance to stay cold.

Get home and put it away as quickly as possible. Make food shopping your last stop before home. Put groceries away as soon as you arrive home.

Storing Foods at Home

Think time and temperature (and always clean). For best quality, use foods soon after buying them. As a general rule, foods should be stored in the home as they were stored at the supermarket, until they are opened. *Appendix 1 has specific recommendations about storage times and temperatures.*

In general, remember to:

Check food labels before you store foods. Don't assume that all canned foods are pantry foods; some need to be refrigerated, even before opening. Different brands may have different requirements. For example, some grated

Parmesan cheese must be refrigerated, but not all.

Use older foods first: "first on the shelf, first out." Put newer purchases behind older purchases. If possible, all foods should be visible so that they're not forgotten.

Store foods in clean areas. Keep pantry, refrigerator, and freezer shelves clean. Make sure you use only clean containers to store flour, sugar, and other dry goods.

The best pantry storage is cool (between 50°F and 60°F; at least below 85°F), dry, dark, and clean. At higher temperatures, foods lose their nutritional and taste quality faster, but they may still be safe to eat. Damaged containers and mold are signs of unsafe foods. Use thermometers to periodically check temperatures.

Store foods away from stoves, ovens, or other heat sources. Heat reduces the shelf life of foods.

Keep cans, jars, and other shelf goods dust-free. Dust may be pressed into canned or jar foods as they are opened. Rinse cans and jars before opening them.

Are any foods sticky? Their packaging may be leaking, or another food may have leaked onto them. Although leaking honey or syrup is not dangerous, it may attract insects. If a canned food is leaking, it may be dangerous. Notify your local health department or return it to the store so they can notify the manufacturer. If you are not sure what the leak is, do not risk tasting the food; discard it so that people and pets will not consume it. One of the best ways to discard it is in a garbage disposal.

Keep the refrigerator set so the temperature is between 34°F and 40°F. If you open your refrigerator frequently or leave it open for a long time, the temperature will rise. To allow the cold air to circulate freely, do not crowd or stack food. Putting large amounts of very hot food in the refrigerator will raise the temperature slightly for a short time, but it is safer than letting foods cool slowly outside the refrigerator. In general, your refrigerator should be as cold as possible without freezing your leafy vegetables or milk.

Store eggs in their protective carton inside the refrigerator. They don't last as long in the refrigerator doors where the temperatures are warmer and they are not as protected.

Freezer temperatures should be below 0°F. All freezer storage recommendations are based on this temperature. It is hard to keep the freezer compartment of a refrigerator at this temperature. Freezer compartments in refrigerators are meant for short-term storage of frozen foods—a week or two. Chest and upright freezers can hold lower temperatures for

Food Dating

"Sell by" dates give the last date that a food should be sold. It can be stored at home for a "reasonable" time. Purchase dated packages only if the "sell by" date has not expired.

"Use by" and "Best if used by" dates tell you how long products will maintain top quality in your home. Depending on the food and if it has been stored properly, it will likely be safe beyond this date.

The "pack" date is when the food was manufactured, processed, or packaged.

38

longer-term storage of frozen foods. Freezers operate most efficiently when full, but keep some space between packages to allow the cold air to circulate.

Package and label food appropriately before you store it. In general, store foods in clean, air-tight, moisture-proof containers or packaging. Label all home-frozen and home-canned foods with the contents and dates. Label all foods you plan to keep for longer than 2 weeks with the purchase date.

Store fresh meats, poultry, and seafoods that will be used soon after purchasing on plates on lower refrigerator shelves. This reduces the chance that they will drip onto other foods, which is important because raw juices often contain bacteria. Otherwise store in the freezer.

Do not store any foods underneath the kitchen sink or any other cabinets that have pipes. Foods stored in these cabinets can attract insects and rodents through openings that are almost impossible to seal completely. Also, leakage from the pipes can damage food products and their containers.

39

Store foods away from cleaning and pest control supplies. Keep the poison control number for your area on your phone, just in case.

If you find a food that should have been refrigerated sitting on the pantry shelf (it happens to everyone), discard it.

If a food has been kept too long, is moldy, discolored or smelly, don't taste it; discard it. The mold you see is just a small part of the mold. You might say it's the tip of the iceberg. Mold grows deep into food, but you see only the surface. The toxins molds make are under the surface. You can sometimes "save" hard cheeses or breads by cutting the mold out (an inch in every direction), but use the remaining product soon because it will mold quickly. Do not try to "save" soft foods with mold, such as jellies or soft cheeses.

If the power goes out...

Power outages come with winter storms, summer storms, and isolated accidents. When a food storage appliances fail due to a power outage—perishable food is at risk. The length of time that power will be out determines what you can do to reduce loss of perishable refrigerated and frozen food.

Major summer hurricanes can result in long outages for large areas. Combined with hot summer weather, your chances of "saving" food are not good. Everyone will want freezer space, ice, or dry ice; there won't be enough to go around.

For long winter storms, outages may cover large areas and last for several days. Even if it's cold outside, keep your food inside. Exposed to sunlight, food will warm-up, even if the air temperature is cold. Also, outside temperatures change throughout the day. Outside you would also be exposing food to unsanitary conditions and animals.

If you have returned home after an appliance has obviously been off and you cannot judge how long the foods were at a compromised temperature, discard the food. Usually, though, power is out for much shorter times, making it easier for you to protect your investment. Prior planning and know-how help:

If the appliance will be working again within a couple of hours, just leave it closed.

41

A fully stocked freezer will usually keep food frozen for 2 days without power. A half-full freezer will usually keep food frozen for about 1 day. If the freezer is not full, quickly group packages together so they will retain the cold more effectively. Put baked goods and frozen nuts on top, then frozen fruits and vegetables, then meats, seafood, and poultry. That way, drips from meat will not contaminate other foods if they begin to thaw.

If the power will be out for longer than the freezer will "keep its cool," put dry ice in the freezer. (CAUTION: Never touch dry ice with bare hands or breathe its vapors in an enclosed area. Dry ice is frozen carbon dioxide, a gas that settles in low areas and is dangerous to breathe in high concentration.)

Unopened refrigerators can keep food cold for 4 to 6 hours, depending on the temperature of the room. If the power will be out for a longer time, put ice in the refrigerator to keep it cool. A block of ice will stay frozen longer than crushed ice. Put it in a pan to catch the drip.

Once the appliance is working, check your food. Use the following guidelines to decide what to do with the food.

For foods in the freezer:

• If ice crystals are still visible and/or the food feels as cold as if refrigerated, it is safe to refreeze. Raw meats and poultry, cheese, juices, breads, and pastries can be refrozen without substantially compromising quality. Prepared foods, fish, vegetables, and fruits can be refrozen safely, but quality may suffer.

• If the food thawed or was held above 40°F for more than 2 hours, it should generally be discarded because bacteria may multiply to unsafe levels under these conditions. The only foods that should be refrozen are well-wrapped hard cheeses, butter, and margarine, breads and pastries without custard fillings, fruits and fruit juices that look and smell acceptable, and vegetables held above 40°F for less than 6 hours.

• Ice cream and other frozen desserts that have melted cannot be refrozen.

43

• Breads and other foods that will not be cooked should be discarded if they are contaminated with drip from other products, especially meats, poultry, fish, or frozen desserts.

• Foods held in the freezer compartment of a refrigerator may thaw faster than foods held in a full freezer. Check them carefully.

For refrigerated foods:

• Fresh meats, poultry, lunch meats, hotdogs, eggs, milk, soft cheeses, and prepared or cooked foods should be discarded if they have been held above 40°F for more than 2 hours because bacteria can multiply to unsafe levels under these conditions.

• Fresh fruits and vegetables are safe as long as they are still firm and there is not evidence of mold, a yeasty smell, or sliminess.

• Juices, opened containers of vinegar and oil salad dressings, ketchup, pickles, jams and jellies, and well-wrapped hard cheeses are safe as long as there is no evidence of mold growth, and they look and smell acceptable.

• Well-wrapped butter and margarine can usually be kept as long as they do not melt, but should be discarded if rancid odors develop.

Keeping the Kitchen Clean and Safe

Clean all surfaces routinely. Do your best to clean all kitchen equipment and utensils thoroughly (with hot, soapy water) after each use. Dirty equipment can contaminate your food and attract pests. Don't forget your kitchen towels, sponges, and dishcloths; wash them often because bacteria can live in moist areas. Sponges can be cleaned regularly in a dishwasher.

Keep cutting boards clean. If you use a cutting board for meat, poultry, or fish, wash the board thoroughly with hot, soapy water and then rinse with a chlorine bleach solution.

Clean knives safely. Hold them in your hand and wash them with hot, soapy water one at a time after using for any one type of food. Do not put them in a soapy sink with other tableware because you might cut your hand trying to find them in a sinkful of sudsy water.

Clean spills and spatters in microwave ovens after cooking.

Take apart and clean equipment such as food processors and meat grinders as soon as possible after use. Use hot, soapy water on all parts of the equipment that contact food. Follow manufacturer's instructions for submerging equipment in water; electrical connections should remain dry at all times.

Making Up A Sanitizing Solution

Ordinary, inexpensive household chlorine bleach makes one of the most effective household sanitizers. Chlorine bleach solutions are best used after cleaning, because dirt, soap, and food particles can reduce their effectiveness. First clean and rinse, then sanitize.

Use the directions on the container, or follow these recommendations. Use fresh solutions. It is best to make up your solution fresh each day because bleach solutions break down to

Preparing Foods

Proper preparation can greatly reduce contamination of food and the risk of foodborne illness.

Wash your hands. Wash your hands with soapy water for at least 20 seconds before and after you complete tasks and when you move from one food to another. When possible, avoid using your hands to mix food. Keep hands away from your mouth, nose, and hair. Always wash hands thoroughly after using the bathroom, changing diapers or pet litter, blowing

salt water during storage. Putting your solution in a labeled spray bottle makes it easy to use.

Very mild solution for cleaning refrigerator and freezer surfaces: 1 teaspoon chlorine bleach in 1 quart of water

Solution for general kitchen use on cutting boards, sinks, and other utensils: 2 teaspoons chlorine bleach in 1 quart of water

After using a bleach sanitizing solution, rinse with clean water, wipe with a paper towel, and allow to air dry.

your nose, smoking, taking medications, or handling pets.

Do not prepare food when you have an infectious disease or infection. Cover any cuts or sores on your hands and lower arms with a bandage to protect you and the food or wear latex gloves. If cuts are infected, do not prepare food. Never cough or sneeze over food.

Wash lids of cans before opening to keep dirt from getting into food. Also, clean the blade of the can opener (the dirtiest half inch in your kitchen!) after each use. Otherwise, some food will stay on the blade and cross-contaminate other foods.

Thoroughly rinse poultry, seafood, fruits, and vegetables in cold running water before cooking. Use a scrub brush on firm fruits and vegetables or shells of shellfish. Peel, if necessary, after rinsing. Dirt, insects, pesticides, and contaminants from handling are on the surfaces of fresh fruits and vegetables. Clean and sanitize the sink when you are finished.

Follow instructions on product labels. Many products specify, "Refrigerate after opening" or "Do not refreeze."

Use equipment properly. Learn how to use a thermometer to correctly judge internal temperatures *(page 21)*.

Cooking Foods

Always cook foods thoroughly. This is the most reliable way to destroy disease-causing bacteria, viruses, parasites, and molds.

Cook foods to a temperature above 140°F to destroy most disease-causing agents. Appendix 1 gives recommended internal temperatures for cooking meats and poultry, visual cues for cooking eggs, and recommendations for home-canned foods. Other foods are cooked to meet taste and texture standards.

Use reliable recipes. Recipes tell you what to do and how to do it. Reliable recipes are detailed enough to ensure safe cooking. For example, meat should be marinated overnight in the refrigerator in a non-metallic container, not in a metal pan at room temperature. Each year people invent new ways to cook food. Some just don't work. For example, a cook once suggested poaching fish in the dishwasher. However, the fish can end up with detergent residue. When you aren't sure about a recipe, call an expert for advice *(see listing on page 115).*

Cook foods at the right oven temperature. Roast meats and poultry at 325°F or above. At very low oven temperatures bacteria may grow to toxic levels before "real" cooking begins.

Cook meats, poultry, and seafood completely without interruption. Partial cooking can permit bacteria to continue growing during storage. "Finish-up cooking" may not "finish off" the disease-causing bacteria, parasites, and viruses.

It's OK to cook most frozen meats, poultry, fish, casseroles, and vegetables while they are still

Is It Still Safe?

Q *After breakfast, I ran some errands. I returned home at noon and discovered that the milk carton had been sitting on the table since I left at 9. Should I throw it out or put it immediately into the refrigerator?*

A Milk will keep at room temperature 4 to 5 hours. But, unless the milk was very fresh, it may be starting to sour. "Turned" milk won't hurt you; you can use it in cooking, if you

frozen. Allow 50 percent more cooking time, though. For example, if you normally bake your casserole for 50 minutes in a 350°F oven, bake a frozen one for 75 minutes. Cooking large pieces of frozen meats or frozen whole chickens and turkeys is not recommended, however, because the outside may dry out before the inside is done. Smaller pieces of meat, especially frozen hamburgers or fish fillets, cook well when frozen. It's better to cook vegetables frozen than to thaw them first.

If you want to use a marinade after it's been in contact with meat, poultry, or fish, bring it to a

wish. Refrigerate it immediately, if you plan to keep it.

Q *The sliced ham I bought yesterday has an iridescent film. Did it spoil that quickly?*
A It is not spoiled. The iridescence on cooked ham is harmless. Ham has high fat and water contents. When these liquids ooze out they reflect light, just like oil on a puddle or wet road.

full boil for at least one minute. The marinade can then be safely used as a sauce for the final dish. And then, brush the sauce only on cooked surfaces using a clean brush.

Do not taste partially cooked foods, including meat, poultry, seafood, or eggs. Refrain from tasting other uncooked foods with raw eggs, including cookie doughs and cake batters.

Cook in clean, made-for-cooking utensils.

Organize preparation times so that all foods for a meal are ready at the same time to avoid holding foods at room temperature prior to serving.

When microwave cooking, heat evenly and thoroughly. Microwave cooking is convenient. To safely prepare or thaw foods in a microwave oven, allow time for even heat penetration. Generally, smaller amounts cook more evenly than larger amounts. Also, uniform products are easier to cook safely. For example, stuffing for chicken or turkey should be cooked separately and not in the bird. Also, do not can foods in a microwave oven.

The following guidelines will help you to safely use your microwave oven. Also, consult your user's guide or a good, current microwave cookbook for information.

• Glass cookware, glass ceramic cookware, and waxed paper are safe for microwave cooking. Before using other types of containers, wraps, or paper products, check to be sure that they are approved for use in the microwave oven. Improper materials may melt, burn, or contain chemicals that can migrate into food during cooking.

• Try to work with smaller, uniform pieces of food to allow even heating. Remove bones from large pieces of meat because these can shield food from thorough cooking. Trim fat.

• Completely defrost frozen food before cooking in a microwave oven. Having frozen and thawed portions in the same food will lead to uneven cooking. Once a food is thawed in the microwave, finish cooking immediately.

• Cover foods with lids or vented plastic wrap that doesn't touch the food. This keeps steam in contact with the food for thorough cooking and prevents surface "sweating".

• Use medium (50 percent power) settings for large cuts of meat or poultry. This allows the whole product to cook thoroughly without drying out some parts.

• Use a rotating microwave pad or rotate foods manually several times during microwaving. Stir liquids several times during heating.

• If your microwave oven has a temperature probe, use it to cook foods to uniform internal temperatures *(see Appendix 1)*. In addition, for meats and poultry check that there is no blood, the juices run clear, and the flesh separates easily from the bones. The internal temperatures for reheated foods should reach over 165°F in all areas immediately after cooking. Take several measurements (at least three) throughout the center region or the thickest portion of the largest piece. If the food is a mixture of solids and liquids, such as a stew, determine the temperature of the largest solid piece. The probe should not contact bone, metal, glass, or any of the packaging material.

• Observe all standing times for microwaved foods. It is part of the cooking time. Consult oven manufacturer's instructions or another current, reliable cookbook.

Allow your slow cookers time to cook. Slow cookers work slowly at low temperatures between 170°F and 280°F. The direct heat from the pot, lengthy cooking, and steam created within the tightly-covered container combine to destroy bacteria. Slow cookers generally take over 2 hours to heat food to bacteria-killing temperatures. The best foods for slow cooking are soups, stews, chili, spaghetti sauce, and similar foods that contain a lot of liquid. To ensure uniform and thorough cooking:

• Use small pieces of meat or poultry. Use refrigerated, not frozen pieces, and keep them in the refrigerator until you are ready to add them to the pot. Large pieces may not cook quickly enough to be safe.

• Fill cookers at least half full, but no more than two thirds full.

• Vegetables cook more slowly than meats, so put them in first—on the bottom and around the sides. Then add meat and cover with liquid.

• Always cook with the lid on. Remove it only to stir or check for doneness.

• If your cooker has more than one setting, use the high setting to bring the liquid to a boil. Then use the setting called for in your recipe. It should be at least 170°F. Once it is done, food will stay safe in the cooker as long as it is operating.

• Reheating refrigerated leftovers in a slow cooker takes too long to get foods out of the

Plastic or Wood?
The Cutting Board Controversy

Should you choose (and use) a plastic or wooden cutting board? Although one laboratory's research suggests that wooden cutting boards are safer than plastic, more recent research has confirmed that plastic is safer for raw foods and cooked meats, poultry or seafood. If you do use a wooden cutting board for meat, poultry, or seafood, use a different board for cutting other foods. This will pre-

danger zone. You can hold reheated food on top of the stove or in the microwave or in a slow cooker for serving.

• As with all electrical appliances, do not leave home when they are on. Do not leave the cooker plugged in when it is not in use.

Serving Foods

Keep hot foods hot, cold foods cold, and everything clean. Serve foods as soon after preparation as possible.

Use clean dishes and utensils to serve food. Dishes and utensils should be washed with

vent cross contamination of bread or produce with bacteria from meat, poultry or seafood.

Whichever type you choose, clean it in hot, soapy water after each use. Sanitize it after cutting meat, poultry, or fish (see page 46 for sanitizing directions). Once cutting boards become excessively worn or develop hard-to-clean grooves, it's best to replace them.

hot, soapy water before using for serving. Serve grilled foods on a clean plate, not the one that held raw meat, poultry, or fish.

Select serving utensils that are intended for food, easy to use, and clean. Wooden utensils are harder to clean than plastic or metal. Wooden chopsticks, toothpicks, and skewers are intended for a single use. Plastic utensils develop cracks that are hard to clean, so use them once. Heavier plastics can be cleaned effectively between uses. Supply easy-to-use serving utensils on buffet lines to keep people from using their fingers.

Use ceramic containers and dishes that are intended for use with food. Some older or decorative ceramic containers and glassware contain toxic lead that can leach into food or beverages.

Keep cooked food at room temperature for no more than 2 hours. Foods held warm on steam tables or in chafing dishes (above 140°F) are usually safe for about 4 hours. Here are some hints for keeping foods safe during serving:

• Keep foods covered when possible to keep them as hot as possible.

58

- Don't add fresh food to food that has been out, unless all of the food will be used in 2 hours. For example, if a buffet was set up at 11:30, new food can be added only if the buffet will finish by 1:30. Instead, bring out a new container; it looks more attractive, too.
- If you are not sure how much food will be eaten, divide it into two or three smaller serving containers and replace the food more frequently.
- Watch to be sure that people do not mishandle food. Using the same utensil for serving several different foods or picking up foods with fingers are common ways of contaminating foods.
- Serving utensils should never be used for tasting.

Leftovers

Keep it safe the second time around. Consider any cooked meat, poultry, seafood, vegetable, or other cooked product a leftover, if it is not served immediately. If handled and stored properly, leftovers can be enjoyed at a later meal or snack.

Food left on individual dinner plates or other "tasted" food should be discarded after a meal. Food that contains even a small amount of saliva from a fork or spoon is contaminated. Even bacteria from your own mouth can grow on food and make you sick when you consume it later if the bacteria have been allowed to multiply. Also, food that has been on a dinner plate may have become contaminated by other foods on that plate.

Safe Handling and Serving of Baby Foods

Baby foods in a jar. Feeding baby directly from a jar introduces bacteria from your baby's mouth, to the spoon, and back into the food. This bacteria can then multiply and may cause diarrhea, vomiting, or other symptoms of foodborne illness if fed to baby at a later feeding. Instead, transfer a small amount of food from a jar to a feeding dish. If your baby needs more, use a clean spoon to transfer more food to the feeding dish. Return the cap to an opened jar of baby food and refrigerate for up to 3 days. Likewise, discard any extra formula that your baby does not drink.

Guidelines for handling leftovers:

• Refrigerate or freeze leftover foods as soon
  after cooking as possible, preferably within
  30 minutes. If food is still very hot, cool it
  quickly in an ice water bath before storing.
  To make an ice water bath, fill a clean sink
  with a mixture of ice and water. Put food in
  a container and submerge it in the water.
  For example, a pot of soup can be lowered

Home-made baby foods. If you choose to make
your own baby foods, make them fresh. Don't
just purée leftovers, because these foods are
more likely to be contaminated than freshly
cooked foods. Also, leftovers may contain sea-
sonings that your baby doesn't need.
Sanitation is extremely important when making home-made baby food. Be sure that foods
are cooked thoroughly, surfaces and equipment are clean, and storage containers are
spotless. Refrigerate or freeze foods immediately after preparation. Use refrigerated foods
within 2 days. Always thaw frozen food in the
refrigerator.

61

into several inches of water and the contents stirred until it cools slightly.

- Store leftovers in clean, shallow, tightly
covered containers. Shallow containers
(2 inches deep) help foods cool more
quickly. It's a good idea to transfer leftover
soups or stews from a large pot to smaller,
more shallow containers. For foods that will
be reheated in a microwave oven, use
microwavable containers.

- Cut roasts into slices of 3 inches thick or
less and take the poultry meat off the car-
cass before storing, since large, dense foods,
such as a whole roasted turkey or beef
roast, do not cool quickly. It is especially
important to chill these foods quickly to
keep bacteria from multiplying.

- Store leftovers in the refrigerator or freezer.
Even foods that were originally stored on
pantry shelves belong in the refrigerator or
freezer after opening or cooking. For example, uncooked rice is usually stored in a
pantry. Once cooked, store it in the refrigerator or freezer. Store potatoes that have
been baked in the refrigerator until used.
Leaving food on a table or in an oven to eat

later gives bacteria the time and environment to grow.

- Store cooked food on shelves located above raw items in the refrigerator to prevent contamination from drips or falling food particles.
- Use leftovers quickly. *Appendix 1 gives some storage times and temperatures for leftovers.*
- Refrigerate or freeze leftover poultry and stuffing separately.
- Bring leftover soups, gravies, and sauces to a boil. Cover other leftovers and reheat them to 165°F to destroy bacteria that may have grown. Foods that have been improperly stored or otherwise mishandled will not necessarily be made safe by reheating. Some leftover foods are often eaten cold, such as meats for sandwiches or pizza, making it even more important to follow storage guidelines.
- If reheating in a microwave oven, cover the dish to retain heat and reduce moisture loss. Let stand a minute or two after microwaving to allow heat to penetrate evenly. Check temperature in three places with a thermometer. It should reach 165°F.

• In general, leftovers should be reheated only once.

Handling Raw Meat and Poultry

You may have noticed a special label with "Safe Handling Instructions" on a package or ground beef or chicken thighs the last time

What Can I Take for Lunch?

Q *I've seen several pre-packed lunches at the grocery store. Can I store them in my desk drawer (or in my child's locker) until lunch time?*

A Many of the lunches contain luncheon meats that require refrigeration. Check the package carefully for instructions. Pre-packed foods sold from refrigerated cases usually need to be refrigerated during storage.

Q *I want milk for lunch, but we do not have it available in our vending machines. I don't have a thermos. What else can I do?*

A Try the shelf-stable, individual serving milks. These are usually sold in the packaged juice section of the grocery store. If you like your milk cold, you can freeze a container overnight, and it will thaw by lunchtime, keeping the rest of your lunch cold, too. Or, serve the milk over ice.

you shopped. In fact, these instructions are required to be on all raw or partially cooked meat and poultry products. *(See page 67.)* Meat and poultry require special handling because they contain naturally-occurring bacteria that often cause illness when mishandled or cooked improperly

Storing and thawing. Safe storing and thawing of meat, poultry, and seafood can prevent foodborne illness. Store these perishable foods at refrigerator temperatures of 40°F and below to slow bacterial growth. Freezer temperatures of 0°F stop bacterial growth.

Thawing meat, poultry, and fish in the refrigerator or microwave oven helps prevent bacterial growth. Never thaw meat, poultry, seafood, or other perishable foods on the countertop because food defrosts from the outside inward. If left to thaw on a counter at room temperature, bacteria can multiply to dangerous levels on the product's surface before the inside completely thaws.

Thawing in the microwave is another safe option, but foods must be cooked immediately after defrosting.

Keep bacteria from spreading. Clean all surfaces, including your hands, after contact with these raw products. This prevents the spread of bacteria from raw meat, poultry, and seafood to other foods that may not be cooked, and utensils used for other foods.

Cook thoroughly. Thorough cooking is the best protection against foodborne illness. Meat and poultry should be cooked to proper temperatures to ensure bacteria are destroyed. *See Appendix 1 for safe endpoint temperatures for food prepared at home.*

Store leftovers promptly. To keep bacteria from multiplying in cooked meat, poultry, and seafood products, don't let them sit out at room temperature for more than 2 hours. Leftovers should be stored in the refrigerator or freezer promptly. Divide large quantities and place into small, shallow containers. This also applies to large pieces of meat and poultry, which should be deboned and divided into smaller serving sizes for safe storage. In addition, remove stuffing from poultry or other stuffed meats and refrigerate in separate containers.

Safe Handling Instructions

This product was prepared from inspected and passed meat and/ or poultry. Some food products may contain bacteria that could cause illness if the product is mishandled or cooked improperly. For your protection, follow these safe handling instructions.

Keep refrigerated or frozen. Thaw in refrigerator or microwave.

Keep raw meat and poultry separate from other foods. Wash working surfaces (including cutting boards), utensils, and hands after touching raw meat or poultry.

Cook thoroughly.

Keep hot foods hot. Refrigerate leftovers immediately or discard.

67

Safe Food for You and Your Family

68

Chapter 3

Away From Home

Most of us consume over half of the food we eat away from home. Some of that food comes from restaurants, vending machines, and other prepared food vendors. But many foods are prepared and packaged at home and eaten somewhere else—usually at school or work. All of the rules of food safety hold here. Mother Nature does not take a lunch break!

Packing Meals From Home

Be sure your lunch bag, box, cooler, or case is clean inside. Always discard leftovers at the end of the meal or day and clean the container inside and out.

Wrap food well to protect it from dirt and drips.

Refrigerate perishable foods, if possible. If you don't have access to a refrigerator, choose foods that are less perishable. Peanut butter and processed cheese are old favorites.

69

Canned meats and fish work, too. Single serving units are just the right size, especially if you cannot refrigerate leftovers. If you can keep your lunch cold, you have a greater range of choices. Remember to check "use by" dates. Use deli meats within 1 to 2 days of purchase and prepacked processed meats and poultry within 3 to 5 days of opening.

Prepare your lunch the night before and store it in the refrigerator to help start the day at the right temperature. If you pack a frozen drink or a reusable freeze-pack with your lunch—or freeze your sandwich—it is more likely to stay at the right temperature. (Sandwiches made with mayonnaise do not freeze well because the mayonnaise separates. That's a taste and texture problem, not a safety problem.) And add the lettuce, tomato, or other veggies just before eating the sandwich. (They don't freeze well either.)

Keep your packaged meal in the coolest possible place. At the very least, keep it away from radiators or sunny windows.

For hot foods, use wide-mouth thermos containers. Rinse the container with very hot water so that it starts out hot. Then add very hot food (165°F or greater) to the thermos. Be sure to check the seal around the stopper to make sure that it fits tightly. Properly packed, your thermos-protected food will keep at a safe, appetizing temperature for 4 hours or so.

If you are packing leftover soup, stew, casseroles, or other home-prepared foods, keep them cold and reheat thoroughly in a microwave oven at work. Or pack them in a thermos (see above).

Wash all fruit carefully before packing it into your lunch. It is harder to wash fruit away from home.

Picnics

It's just as important at picnics to follow the rules of food safety: keep hot foods hot, cold foods cold, and everything clean. It may take more planning, but your efforts will be rewarded by a safe food event!

Prepare cold foods far in advance. This allows food to chill thoroughly before packing and transporting.

71

Pack cold foods directly from the refrigerator into a well-insulated cooler. Layer the cooler with crushed ice or blue ice packs to maintain a temperature below 40°F.

When possible, use two coolers for cold foods. The beverage and snack cooler can be opened

Insulated Coolers vs Refrigerators— The Cold Truth

Wanting to know what products are the "smartest" and easiest to use, the announcer asked several audience members what they thought. Most mentioned computers. One man, though, said his thermos was the smartest. The announcer didn't expect such a low-technology answer. He looked at his viewer and said, "But it just keeps food hot or cold." The man looked right back at him and asked, "Yes, but how does it know which one?"

Coolers, like thermos containers, are insulators. They keep temperatures from changing quickly. That means that, if you pack a food hot, it will help keep it hot. If you pack a food cold, it will help keep it cold. The better the

frequently without affecting the cooler with meats, salads, and other cold perishables.

Pack foods in reverse-use order. First foods packed are the last ones used—and they're on the bottom.

insulation, the longer the temperature is maintained. To work, the cooler must remain sealed. If you open and close it, or if it has a poor seal or a hole, it cannot hold temperature effectively. Also, coolers work best when they are full.

Refrigerators circulate cooled air. Unlike coolers, they can reduce temperatures of foods. The process of removing heat from foods requires energy. We don't have to "plug in" coolers, but we do have to supply energy to refrigerators. When the power goes out, a refrigerator or freezer becomes a cooler, and the food cannot be stored in it for a long time.

Pack raw meats, poultry, or seafood on the bottom of the insulated chest. This reduces the risk of them dripping on other foods.

If possible, pack coolers until they're full. A full cooler will stay cold longer than one that is partially filled.

Keep coolers in the coolest, shadiest place possible while picnicking. Cover them with a light-colored blanket to protect them from sunlight. Try to transport your coolers in the passenger area of your car; it's cooler than the trunk.

If you don't have an insulated cooler, take less perishable foods. Examples include fresh fruits, hard cheese, canned meats or fish, peanut butter, breads, crackers, etc.

Do not partially cook foods before transporting them. Partial cooking may not destroy bacteria, allowing them to multiply in the interim. It is okay to reheat cooked food on site. For example, you may roast your chicken thoroughly at home and rewarm it, brushed with barbecue sauce, on a grill at the picnic.

Keep vegetables or fruits intended for grilling separate from raw meats. Someone may come along and eat some of those delicious-looking raw items. You don't want them to be contaminated with drip from the raw meats or fish.

Carry hot foods in well-insulated containers. And pack hot foods separate from cold foods. to keep them above 140°F.

Bring moist towelettes to clean hands before and after handling foods.

In hot weather (above 85°F) food should not sit out for longer than one hour. After one hour service time, perishable food should be discarded.

Barbecues

Whether as a part of a picnic or for variety at home, barbecuing signals fun. All the normal food safety rules hold, but you'll also want to consider the following:

Precook large cuts of meat or poultry in the oven or microwave, and then finish cooking them immediately on the grill. Larger cuts of poultry and/or beef don't always barbecue well, because the outside tends to burn before the

inside is really cooked. But you can get barbecue flavor by grilling them for the last 30
minutes.

**Use a separate platter to carry raw meats to the
grill and cooked meats from the grill.** Or wash
the platter thoroughly between uses. Do not
let drippings from platters holding raw meat,
poultry, or fish fall onto other foods.

**Do not use utensils that were used to handle raw
foods for handling cooked products.** For example, the cooking brush used for spreading the
barbecue sauce on the raw cuts should not be
used again as the last step for glazing the
ready-to-eat food.

**Use a thermometer to check doneness for large
pieces of meat or poultry.** Do not taste meat to
determine if it is properly cooked and then
put it back on the grill.

Smoking Foods

Smoking is a grilling technique that slow
cooks meat while adding flavor. If you have
the right equipment, it can be just the right
way to cook foods for a longer family outing
or small reunion. All of the leftover rules still

hold. Since the food is likely to be outside, serve it for no longer than an hour in warm weather.

• Pile about 50 briquets of high-quality charcoal in the center of the smoker (covered grill). When they are hot and covered with gray ash, push them into two piles. Center a pan of water between the two piles. (Don't burn your fingers!) Mesquite or hickory chips give additional flavor to the smoke. Using dry chips at the start creates a fast smoke. Wet them later for sustained heat. Center the food over the water pan and close the lid.

• Keep the grill vents open. The temperature in the smoker should be maintained between 250 to 300°F for safety. Add about ten coals every 1 to 2 hours during the smoking process.

• Beef is done when it reaches an internal temperature of 160°F. Pork should reach 170°F, and poultry should reach 180°F.

• Large, whole, fatty fish such as dressed salmon is done when it reaches 145°F. Fish has a tendency to stick to the grill, so grease the grill and the fish before smoking it.

Camping and Backpacking

Lack of refrigeration is the biggest problem for camp foods. Lack of safe water is the second biggest problem.

Knowing your camp area is important. Is water available? Can you have a campfire? How can you safely dispose of garbage? Keep these important considerations in mind:

Don't take any more ice-requiring foods than you can use early in the trip. Even the newer insulated carriers can only keep food refrigerator-cold for a day. For later in your trip, when you'll need food that doesn't need to be kept cold, bring canned foods, peanut butter, cereals, and dried foods. If you have a source of safe drinking water available, dried foods score a plus—they are lighter to carry!

You can take bottled water for drinking or mixing with food—but it's heavy. Otherwise, you can boil stream or river water for 15 minutes (covered); allow to stand for 30 minutes to let mud and debris settle; dip out water and strain it through a clean cloth before using. Or use commercial purification tablets, following all instructions carefully.

78

If you catch fish when camping, clean and wash them thoroughly, then cook immediately. Do not try to store fish for later unless you have plenty of ice.

Help your cooler stay cool. Wrap your cooler in newspapers or cover it with a sleeping bag, and then put it in the shade.

For outdoor cooking after dark, check any meat (especially hamburgers) with a thermometer. Everything looks done in the dark.

Bringing Home the Catch

Bring your fish and shellfish home safely by following these tips:

Keep fish cold. The colder the temperature, the slower the rate of spoilage. Stuff the body cavity of large fish with ice immediately after gutting. Cut very large fish into pieces small enough to fit into your cooler.

You may want to prepare fish completely by removing scales, heads, and intestines, or by filleting them—so they will be freezer-ready when you get home. At the very least remove the heads or gills and the intestines and rinse well. Large fish should be bled and gutted immediately upon capture.

At your destination, unpack your catch. Rinse fish under cold, running water. Put shellfish in the refrigerator as described in Appendix 1. If you are not planning to cook them right away, package and freeze fish or shellfish for future use. The sooner fish and shellfish are frozen after harvest, the longer they will be safe to eat.

Never thaw fish and shellfish at room temperature. Place the package in cold, running water, or leave it in your refrigerator overnight.

Freezing Fresh Fish and Shellfish:

Freeze fish by coating them with a glaze of lemon juice and gelatin.

- Measure 1/4 cup of bottled lemon juice into a pint container, and fill the rest of the container with water.
- Dissolve one packet of unflavored gelatin in 1/2 cup of the mixture.

- Heat the remaining liquid to boiling; then stir the dissolved gelation mixture into the boiling liquid.
- Cool to room temperature.

- Dip the fillet or fish in the liquid; allow it to drain for several seconds when you lift it out.
- Wrap the fish tightly in a heavy, protective plastic film designed for freezer storage. Using a high-quality freezer wrap is very important. Label and date the finished package. Freeze at 0°F as quickly as possible.

Shrimp should be headed and frozen in their shells in freezer containers. After filling the carton, cover the shrimp with ice water, leaving enough head space for the water to expand when frozen (about 1/2 inch).

Scallops should be shucked and frozen in air-tight containers.

Clams and oysters are best frozen in their shells, which makes them easy to shuck with no loss of juices. Otherwise, they can be shucked and frozen in air-tight containers.

Crabs should be cleaned and cooked before freezing. Freeze the meat in the cores and claws, but thaw in the refrigerator before picking the meat out. The quality of the crab meat will be superior to that of meat that is picked while frozen.

Ideally, all frozen fish and shellfish should be used within 2 months for maximum quality. When properly frozen, lean fish such as floun-

Transporting Live Shellfish

Crabs and lobsters. To carry live crabs and lobsters, place 3 to 4 inches of ice in the bottom of the cooler. Cover with waxed cardboard or plastic foam in which holes have been punched. This allows the cold to escape, but keeps the shellfish out of contact with ice or water. Place the shellfish on the cardboard or foam, and cover them with damp burlap. Leave the lid slightly ajar for air circulation. Maintain a temperature of 40° to 50°F. They will be inactive, but they will revive when removed from the cold temperature. Limit holding time to one day. Do not use any crabs or lobsters that die. Live crabs show movement of the legs. Live lobsters show some leg

der, snapper, and trout should maintain quality up to 6 months. Fatty fish such as bluefish, mackerel, and mullet should be used within 3 months. Shrimp, scallops, clams, oysters, and crabs can be stored up to 3 months.

Superchilling is also an excellent way to store fresh fish immediately after catching them.

What you will need:

movement and their tails curl under their bodies and do not hang down when they are picked up.

Oysters and clams. Oysters need to be kept moist, and can be transported in the same way as crabs. Although clams need a drier environment and greater air circulation, they, too, can be successfully carried in this manner or placed on top of ice. Do not place ice on top of clams. Maintain a temperature of 35° to 45°F for both oysters and clams. Limit holding time to 2 to 3 days. Discard any that are not alive when you reach your destination. The shells of live oysters and clams will be tightly closed or will close tightly when tapped.

83

- insulated cooler (the better the insulation, the longer the ice will stay frozen),
- flaked or crushed ice, and
- rock or table salt. (Do not use ice that is rough or jagged because it will cut the fish flesh.)

What to do:

In a separate container, make a salt/ice mixture, using about 1/2 pound of salt for every 5 pounds of ice.

If the cooler does not have a drain, first place a rack in the bottom to keep the seafood out of any water that may accumulate from melting ice.

Line the cooler with 3 to 4 inches of flaked or crushed ice.

Layer the fish in the cooler, covering each layer with the salt/ice mixture. Eviscerated fish should be unwrapped and the body cavities filled with ice. Dressed fish and shucked shellfish should be wrapped in heavy, clear plastic film; shrimp should be headed, left in the shells and wrapped in heavy, clear plastic film.

When the cooler is filled, top with a generous layer of ice and close securely. Also close the drain plug.

Place the cooler in a cool, shady section of your car, not in the trunk.

Drain off melted water at night and add more ice. On longer trips, you may need to add more salt.

Holiday and Company Meals

So, everyone's coming to your house. You'll be preparing food for more people than usual. And maybe you have guests with special food safety needs—someone undergoing cancer therapy, someone "older" or "younger" or perhaps pregnant. You're probably stretching your food storage seams to bursting. What you need is a food safe plan.

First, develop your menu. Next, determine whether you need to alter your menu to meet the needs of your guests who have a greater risk of foodborne illness. Then, begin your shopping and preparation plans. Here's an example using a traditional holiday meal:

85

A Traditional Thanksgiving Menu:
Raw Vegetables with Herb Dip
Turkey and Stuffing, with Gravy
Squash Custard Casserole
Mashed Potatoes • Green Beans
Fruit Salad
Dinner Rolls
Pumpkin Mousse with
Pecan Meringue Topping

Food-safe Considerations. Instead of serving raw vegetables with dip, consider stuffing celery sticks or topping vegetable slices with dip to make an attractive tray with individual servings. Many people bite and re-dip, adding their saliva (with bacteria) to the dip. Unless served over ice, dips tend to sit at room temperature for long periods, allowing growth of bacteria.

Instead of serving turkey and stuffing, consider turning the stuffing into dressing. Just add a little more liquid and cook it in a separate pan for the last 45 minutes or so that the turkey is roasting. It's safer because the bacteria on the inside of the turkey won't contaminate it. *If you do choose to stuff the bird, review the information on page 89.*

Clean vegetables thoroughly in cold, running water. Use a clean scrub brush for vegetables with thicker skins. Cook just before serving.

If you prepare a vegetable casserole in advance, cook it completely in a shallow container (no more than 2 inches deep) before refrigerating it. Then you can reheat to 165°F before serving. If you plan to reheat in a microwave oven, cook the casserole in a microwave-safe serving dish.

Wash all fruits thoroughly in cold, running water. Peel fruits with a clean knife. Mix with a clean utensil, not your hands (but keep your hands clean all the time).

If your pumpkin mousse contains uncooked eggs, rethink your recipe. Look for a recipe (or adapt your own recipe) that requires the eggs to be thoroughly cooked for the custard portion of the mousse. And consider using whipped cream instead of whipped egg whites for the mousse. The meringue may also be a problem since it contains egg whites that are not usually thoroughly cooked. Instead, make firm meringue "dollops" to top your mousse. These can be prepared the night before and stored in an airtight container in the refrigerator until the mousse is served. For an even safer option, consider the traditional traditional pumpkin pie or a pumpkin custard. These options are thoroughly cooked, reducing your risk of foodborne disease.

Shopping and Preparation. All food safety rules hold here. Remember these general tips:

You will probably need extra refrigerator and freezer room for holiday and other special meals. Plan early to use up foods that you are storing. Some foods can be removed from the refrigerator for several days and returned for longer storage, such as raw fruits and vegetables, ketchup, mustard, commercial oil-and-vinegar salad dressings, pickles, and hard cheeses. Other foods—meats, eggs, soft cheeses, luncheon meats, yogurt, custard or cream-type pies, and cakes with egg-white or cream-cheese based icings—should be kept refrigerated for their entire storage period.

Counter tops, utensils, and sinks should be clean before you start food preparation. Store any clean dishes that are drying, and wash any soiled ones before you start. Then clean off the counter top with hot, soapy water, rinse, and dry. This will help reduce the chance of contaminating fresh foods as you work with them and will make sink space available for washing fruit, vegetables, and other foods as you prepare them.

If you have "cooked ahead" and frozen foods, reheat them to 165°F without thawing.

Turkey requires care from its purchase to the time to store, cook, serve, and use leftovers. See "Turkey Tips" on page 90 and the following instructions for stuffing.

Stuffing a Turkey

Don't try to save time by pre-stuffing. Dry stuffing ingredients can be prepared the day before, tightly covered, and left at room temperature. The perishables (mushrooms, oysters, cooked celery and onions, broth, etc.) should be refrigerated. Combine ingredients just before stuffing the fully thawed and rinsed turkey.

Stuff lightly. Stuffing expands when it cooks. You want heat to penetrate evenly. Do not stuff poultry that will be cooked in a microwave oven. It may not cook thoroughly.

Roast your turkey at 325°F until the stuffing reaches 165°F. Use a thermometer to measure this temperature.

Remove stuffing as soon as your turkey is completely cooked. Stuffing left in the turkey can support rapid growth of bacteria. Put the stuffing in a clean casserole or serving dish, and keep it hot in the oven at 200°F until you need it.

More Turkey Tips

Buy frozen turkeys early enough to thaw them safely—1 day in the refrigerator for every 5 pounds of turkey. Microwave-thawing is not a good technique for large birds because it begins to cook them. If you buy your bird pre-stuffed, do not thaw before cooking.

Roast your turkey at 325°F to an internal temperature of 180°F. Roasting the turkey at very low temperatures is not recommended because the turkey might take several hours to reach a high enough temperature to kill bacteria. That means that the bacteria have

**Store any leftover stuffing in a container sepa-
rate from the turkey for up to 2 days.** If the
stuffing is at room temperature for 2 hours or
more, discard it. Reheat leftover stuffing to
165°F to serve.

Food Functions for Club, Community, and Religious Groups

Community and religious group functions
commonly feature "potluck" meals. Also, many
outreach programs for elderly and homeless

more time to grow. You might not be able to
destroy them all during cooking.

Although a time-honored tradition, basting is
not necessary because it cannot penetrate the
turkey. Also opening the oven door frequently
prolongs cooking time.

Do not leave a turkey out for "picking."
Fingers carry bacteria. Put leftovers away as
soon as possible. At least within 2 hours of
cooking, debone the bird and divide the meat
into smaller portions for storage. Freeze what
you will not eat in 2 days.

91

are sponsored by groups that use untrained or minimally trained volunteers. Preparing food for other people is a big responsibility. To keep the "fun" in *fun*ction:

Appoint a person who knows foodservice and food safety to coordinate and supervise the activities. You may already have members who have this experience. If not, call the Health Department, Cooperative Extension Office, or local community college to seek training.

Try to plan so that, as much as possible, the food production is conducted in an approved and licensed kitchen. Although kitchens located in religious and social halls are technically under the Board of Health, they have probably not been inspected. Call your local Health Department for inspection and help. This is especially important if the organization sponsors a home-delivered meal program or supports a homeless shelter.

Follow all standard safety procedures as outlined in "Safe Food at Home" *(pages 25–67)*. Pay careful attention to reducing contamination of food by sick or infected food handlers and keeping food out of the danger zone (40° to 140°F). Reheat all food thoroughly.

Inspect donated food. Be sure that it is at an appropriate temperature. If it is commercially packaged, be sure that the packaging is intact. Be sure that it is "in date."

Cooking for a Crowd

Q *I plan to prepare a large batch of bread pudding for my club luncheon. I want it to be warm when I serve it. Can I make it in the morning, bake it for 30 minutes of the hour baking time, turn off the oven and finish baking it before serving*

A It's never a good idea to partially cook potentially unsafe foods. Because bread pudding contains both eggs and milk, it is potentially hazardous. You may not destroy all the pathogens with this cooking method, and they will have plenty of time to grow while the oven is turned off. Prepare the bread pudding completely the night before and refrigerate it. Reheat it at the luncheon, while you are eating, if possible.

93

Store food in the right containers. Store acidic punches, fruit juices, and soft drinks in food grade plastic, glass, or stainless steel. Do not use galvanized pans or buckets or enamelware for these products. Do not store food in plastic garbage bags or "clean" trash cans.

Provide appropriate cold storage. Refrigerators are the best (and try to keep doors closed as much as possible). You can use insulated coolers for short storage, but use them correctly (page 72).

If you are transporting food, do it right! Always clean the transport area thoroughly. Vehicles used to carry pets, recycling materials, or chemicals (including fertilizers and pesticides) are hard to clean. If in doubt, find another vehicle.

If you are using a caterer, check with your local Health Department about their experiences with the caterer. Be sure that your caterer is licensed and insured. Be your own inspector. Make sure their transport vehicles are sanitary, their hands and utensils clean, and their food at the appropriate temperature.

Food Gifts

Mail-order foods can make excellent gifts, but they need to be checked carefully. Enjoy them as soon as possible. Transport does not improve quality or extend shelf life.

Cooking for a Crowd

Q *I'm in charge of preparing sandwiches for 50 volunteers who will be making house repairs in a limited-resource neighborhood. The workers will take their lunches with them, and there is no refrigeration on-site. What is the safest way to prepare and pack the lunch?*

A Have your group meet and prepare the sandwiches the day before. Chill them overnight, and pack them in a cooler. Reusable freezer-packs will keep them cold. Or, freeze the sandwiches before packing them in the cooler. They will thaw before lunch. Whether you freeze or refrigerate your sandwiches, send the condiments—mayonnaise, lettuce, tomato—separately. Mayonnaise will separate in the freezer. Lettuce and tomato get soggy fast. Mustard can make it through refrigeration or freezing, though.

If foods do not require refrigeration and the packaging is intact, open and enjoy. If foods require refrigeration, check when you open them to be sure that they are very cold to the touch (as if in the refrigerator). If not, call for a replacement. If packages contain dry ice, do

Cooking for a crowd

Q *My committee plans to serve food in a homeless shelter during the week. Most of my committee members will have to drop their food off on their way to work. What's the safest (and easiest) way?*

A Have them prepare their casseroles, soups, or stews ahead of time and freeze them. That way, they can have them ready in the morning before they leave. Left in the refrigerator at the shelter during the day, they can thaw before you bake, cook, or reheat them. If the food has not thawed before cooking, either cook it frozen (takes about 50% longer) or thaw in the microwave oven (if available) and then cook. Remember to check the temperature of the final products or observe them to be sure that the liquid is bubbling.

not touch the dry ice or its wrapping; it is very cold.

If you are making and sending food gifts, select the items carefully and package them securely.

• Select foods that are not potentially unsafe. Do not send home-canned foods in the mail. They can break, leak, or lose their seals.

• Select sturdy foods that will not break or bruise during transport.

• Package foods securely in food wrap. Then select a strong, waterproof box for shipping. Support the food with packaging material—plain popped corn or styrofoam "peanuts" are good.

• Seal the box well to avoid tampering during shipment. Mark the box "PERISHABLE."

• If you are the recipient of a homemade food gift, check it just as you would check a commercial gift.

Childcare Centers

You can learn a lot about food safety in your child's daycare center by observation. Look

97

for the following, and ask questions when you do not see these safety precautions.

- Staff and children wash their hands frequently with soapy water.
- Surfaces, such as table tops used for both play and eating, are washed with soapy water, rinsed, and disinfected after each use.
- Diaper areas are separate from eating and food preparation areas.

Cooking for a Crowd

Q *My club has a soup and sandwich fundraiser each year. We get together the day before to make the soup. This year it soured. What happened?*

A If you cooked your soup in large batches and put it in the refrigerator in big pots, it just did not cool fast enough. The bacteria in it grew overnight and changed the texture and flavor of the soup. Besides spoiling the soup, foodborne illness-causing bacteria could have multiplied to unsafe levels. Next time, divide the soup into shallow containers (2 inches deep) for chilling. Or, make the soup ahead of time, freeze it (again in small batches), and thaw it in the refrigerator the night before. Bring the soup to a boil, stirring frequently, before serving it.

- Children who help prepare foods have clean hands and are well—no runny noses or cuts on their hands. Children are supervised to be sure that they do not taste food while preparing.
- Foods are stored properly.
- Kitchen surfaces are sanitized before any food preparation takes place.
- Foods are thoroughly cooked.
- Leftovers are handled and reheated correctly. Generally, leftovers show poor planning, especially in small facilities with limited storage.
- Medicines are kept away from foods.

Handwashing in Child Daycare Centers
Handwashing is probably the most important factor in preventing spread of infectious disease in child daycare centers. As a parent-observer, watch for child and staff handwashing

- whenever they come in contact with body fluids (blowing noses, etc.)
- after toileting, assisting a child with toileting, or changing diapers
- before handling food and after handling raw meat, poultry or fish

99

- before handling plates, utensils or setting the table
- before and after eating meals and snacks
- after handling pets or other animals
- after play and nap sessions

Teach your child how to wash her or his hands. First wet hands. Then lather up. Rub soapy hands together and around while counting slowing to twenty. One way to do this is to have the child count the number and say his or her whole name. Then rinse. Dry on a clean towel (usually disposable towels in centers).

Chapter 4

Our Food Supply is (Still) Changing

The end of World War I marked the beginning of the modern kitchen. Gas stoves replaced wood- and coal-burning stoves, and the mechanical refrigerator replaced the ice box. The modern kitchen and the modern food market grew up together. Canned, frozen, and packaged foods nudged fresh produce and meats for more and more space in the market. Because these processed foods could be available year-round at very reasonable prices and required less food preparation skill, their share of the plate grew and grew. After World War II, fewer and fewer women stayed home, further increasing the growth of prepared foods which fed hungry families fast.

Safe, abundant food has always been a priority. Smoking and drying have been used to pre-

101

serve food for over 8,000 years. Salt has been used as a food preservative for at least 2,500 years. In comparison, canning, pasteurization, and freezing are about 100 years old. Food additive use began with salting but has increased as other ingredients were found to improve safety and quality of foods.

Food Additives

Almost 3,000 different substances are added to food to improve eating qualities, storage characteristics, nutrient content, cooking or processing, and safety. The most common food additives are sugar, salt, and corn syrup. All chemicals added to food are tested for safety. Pesticides, detergents, and other chemicals that become a part of food during its production are tested just as chemicals that we intentionally add to food. For example, detergents used commercially on food surfaces, must be approved. These tests look specifically for chemicals that can cause birth defects, cancer, or other physical problems. It takes over ten years of testing for approval. This is such an expensive process that very few chemicals—only the most effective ones—are worth the effort.

102

After approval of a food additive, the FDA determines how it can be used in food. Usually additives are approved for use at levels below 1 percent of the highest "no effect" level from animal testing. This means that, if 100 units is the least amount that cause no reaction, only 1 unit or less can be used in food. Additives that caused cancer at any level are not approved. Food producers must use an additive at the lowest effective level, even if using more would be safe.

Although most food additives are "invisible" unless you are a label reader, some have made it into the news.

FD&C Yellow no. 5 is also called tartrazine. It can cause an allergic-type reaction in sensitive individuals. About 1 in every 10,000 Americans is sensitive, and most of them are allergic to aspirin. It is required to be listed as an ingredient on food labels when it is in a food.

Sulfites are chemicals that have been used for centuries as anti-browning agents for dried fruit. About 2 percent of the 9 million people with asthma in the United States are sulfite-

103

sensitive. Recognition of this problem came with extensive use of sulfites on fresh produce in salad bars in the early 1980s. Use of sulfites is not currently allowed on fresh fruits and vegetables, and processed foods and red wines that contain sulfites must be labeled.

Nitrites used in curing ham, bacon and some other processed meats reduce bacterial growth and toxin production. Nitrites have been shown to contribute to production of nitrosamines, potential cancer-causing substances. It is permitted in cured meats because there is no substitute ingredient available, and the risk of bacterial food poisoning is greater than the risk of cancer from nitrosamines. Although nitrite is found naturally in leafy green vegetables, beer and fried bacon contribute more nitrosamines to the diet than all other foods combined.

Pesticides

The Environmental Protection Agency (EPA) is responsible for approving pesticides and other chemicals used for growing foods. Each approved pesticide can be used only for approved foods. This keeps the level of any single pesticide from getting too high in the environment or our food supply.

For pesticide approval, the EPA looks at the same kinds of data used for food additives plus data on occupational exposure. The EPA then sets the amounts that can be safely used. Then the FDA and USDA look for pesticide residues—small amounts present after production of the food. Sampling consistently shows that 96 to 99 percent of tested foods, including imported foods, have lower than required pesticide residues. Actually, pesticide residues in foods are much lower now than they were 25 years ago. Most samples with illegal residues have approved pesticides on the wrong foods. Although pesticide residues are unlikely to exceed allowable levels in the United States, sampling results are not available instantly. It is possible for some violative products to reach consumers. It is unusual though, but when it does, it makes headlines.

New Food Processes

Newer methods of food preservation and food production are making the news now. Older methods of food preservation were usually adapted from extremes of nature—freezing fish in ice, salting fish in evaporated sea water, and drying fish in arid climates. Then we learned about disease-causing bacteria, viruses, parasites, and molds and were able to use our knowledge to control them by canning and pasteurization. This knowledge also told us how freezing, salting, and drying worked and helped us to improve those processes. Now we have extended this control to another process that helps to destroy disease-causing bacteria and parasites—irradiation.

Similarly, we have bred plants for desirable characteristics for hundreds of years. We have improved our production of foods from animals through breeding and improved nutrition. Biotechnology is an extension of these breeding programs.

Food irradiation. Food irradiation is used to preserve foods by destroying bacteria, parasites, and pests and delaying ripening of fruits and vegetables. Legally it's described as a food additive (preservative), but it is easier to describe as a process. Over 40 years of research support use of irradiation as a food preservation method. European food processors irradiate over 28 billion pounds of food each year. The United States has 40 licensed irradiation facilities. Most of these are used to sterilize medical and pharmaceutical supplies, but 16 also irradiate spices for wholesale use and several others irradiate other foods (citrus fruits, tropical fruits, strawberries, tomatoes, mushrooms, potatoes, onions, and poultry).

In irradiation, food is exposed to radiant energy, which is similar to microwaves. The food is put in a closed unit—an irradiator—where it is treated with the energy rays. These rays penetrate the food and its packaging, just the way microwaves would. Most of the energy passes through, but some is retained in the product as heat. The kind of energy used does not make products radioactive.

As with other food additives, the FDA regulates allowed doses. They are set at the lowest level needed for the desired effect. Doses of irradiation approved in the US by the FDA are the most restrictive of the 38 countries that allow irradiation. Low doses control parasites in fresh pork, slow ripening of fruits and vegetables to keep them from spoiling, and control insects in food. Medium doses control

107

bacteria in poultry. High doses control microorganisms in herbs, spices, and teas; this is important because there is not a good way to wash these products.

How can you know whether a food has been irradiated? All irradiated foods—domestic and imported—in the United States must be labeled with a radura *(at left)*. They must also bear the words, "treated by irradiation" or "treated with radiation." Products that contain irradiated ingredients, such as spices, are not required to be labeled.

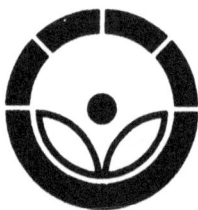

Does irradiation change food? Irradiation causes so few chemical changes in foods that the biggest challenges in regulation are verifying that unlabeled foods have not been irradiated and that labeled foods have received the intended dose. Although some chemicals are formed during irradiation, they are the same chemicals that form during cooking and other common food production processes. As a result of irradiation, disease-causing bacteria and parasites die, making foods safer to eat. In

108

fact, people requiring the safest food—hospital patients with compromised immune systems such as people receiving bone marrow transplants—are routinely given irradiated foods. Nutrient losses in irradiated foods are small and are usually less than nutrient losses during canning, pasteurization, and cooking.

If I buy irradiated food, does it need to be treated differently? Irradiated fruits and vegetables are no different from other foods. You will probably notice that irradiated fruits and vegetables last longer though, because irradiation delays ripening (including potato sprouting) and reduces spoilage by molds, bacteria, and insects. Fresh fruits and vegetables still need to be washed, because they can become contaminated before you buy them. Store them and cook them as you would any untreated produce. For any meats, be sure to purchase product with intact packaging. Bacteria and viruses can contaminate meat and poultry after processing, so all the safe handling and cooking guidelines still hold.

Biotechnology

We have used biotechnology for thousands of years. We have fermented products to make cheeses, yogurt, breads, vinegar, and a variety of beverages. We have bred plants and animals to improve yields and eating characteristics. High-yield rice, pest-resistant grains, and tastier produce are results of biotechnology, as are animals bred to produce leaner meat and more milk. These are older, established examples of biotechnology.

Today's scientists are using the knowledge from these established technologies to develop new plant and animal products. We understand that biological characteristics such as disease resistance or vitamin production are established by the DNA in genes. We can identify which genes are responsible for those specific characteristics. Then we can copy genes from one source and transfer them to another, or we can block a gene to keep it from working. This process, called genetic engineering, is what many people call biotechnology.

Newer biotechnologies are more predictable and efficient. In the older methods, unwanted

110

traits were passed along with desirable ones. That meant that it took many generations to produce the desired product. With newer technologies, the desired product can be produced in a single generation.

The first of the newer generation biotechnology products in the market include the Flavr Savr (Calgene, Inc.) tomato and bST-milk. The Flavr Savr tomato is genetically altered by "turning off" the gene that promotes softening of tomatoes during ripening. That means that the tomato can continue to develop a deep red color and a strong tomato flavor without become too soft. The Flavr Savr tomato can be picked and marketed fully ripe instead of "mature green," making it more flavorful at the plate.

Bovine somatotropin (bST) is a cow hormone. It is needed for milk production. The bST gene can be isolated from cows and grown by special bacteria. When harvested and injected into dairy cows maintained under ideal management conditions, milk production increases by 10 to 25 percent. Here the milk quality does not change; the yield is increased.

Are genetically engineered foods safe to eat?
The FDA currently evaluates each application of biotechnology to animal products such as meat and milk on a case-by-case basis. However, the FDA has determined that plant foods produced through biotechnology are no riskier than foods produced by selective breeding and require no special regulation. Developers of genetically-modified plant foods must determine levels of known naturally occurring toxicants, allergens, and nutrients in the new food; safety of any new substances that are produced; and environmental impacts of the crop. These are the same requirements for traditional plant selective breeding processes.

In both the Flavr Savr tomato and bST-milk, no new components that could cause allergic reactions are introduced. In fact, nothing is added to the tomato. With milk, bST occurs naturally, and supplementation does not increase the level of bST beyond normal ranges or change the nutrient content of milk. In fact, fewer cows are able to produce the milk, resulting in less pollution from animal waste.

112

Current biotechnology applications in plant foods include:

- potatoes and tomatoes resistant to viruses that often reduce crop yields
- engineered bacteria that can produce fertilizer in plants
- "super oats" rich in fiber thought to have a cholesterol-lowering effect
- strawberries and tomatoes with more vitamin C

Potential uses of biotechnology in animal production include:

- use of porcine somatotropin (pST) to increase leanness in pork
- development of vaccines to protect animals from disease
- improvement of growth rates and reduced feed costs in farm animals
- more rapid disease detection

Will genetically engineered food be labeled differently? Most new foods will not require special labels, except under certain circumstances. If a new food has a different nutrient profile, it must be labeled. For example, a new tomato variety with more vitamin C would

113

require a label statement. Also, if a gene from a food that could cause an allergic reaction (such as wheat) is transferred to another food, the new food label must contain a statement. Most foods developed through plant biotechnology, however, have no change in nutritional value or composition of the food. Some new products may carry a descriptive brand name, such as "Flavr Savr" for the new tomato.

Chapter 5

Help!

Help can be a telephone call away. You have resources in your local community. The Health Department and the Cooperative Extension Service can answer many of your questions. Additionally, there are many government and voluntary agencies that provide food safety information.

American Council for Science and Health
(ACSH)
1995 Broadway, 16th Floor
New York, NY 10023-5860
(212) 362-7044

The American Dietetic Association (ADA)
National Center for Nutrition and Dietetics
(NCND)
216 W Jackson Blvd
Chicago, IL 60606-6995
(800) 366-1655

115

American Public Health Association (APHA)
1015 Fifteenth St, NW
Washington, DC 20005
(202) 789-5600

Council for Agricultural Science and Technology
(CAST)
137 Lynn Ave
Ames, IA 50010-7120
(515) 292-2125

Egg Nutrition Center
2301 M St, NW
Washington, DC 20037
(800) 833-EGGS

Drinking Water Hotline
US Environmental Protection Agency
(800) 426-4791

Food Marketing Institute (FMI)
1750 K St, NW
Washington, DC 20006-2394
(202) 452-8444

Food and Nutrition Information Center
National Agricultural Library
Room 304
10301 Baltimore Blvd
Beltsville, MD 20705
(301) 344-3719

Institute of Food Technologists (IFT)
221 N LaSalle St
Chicago, IL 60601
(312) 782-8424

International Association of Milk, Food, and Environmental Sanitarians (IAMFES)
6200 Aurora Ave
Suite 200W
Des Moines, IA 50322-2863
(515) 276-3344 or (800) 369-6337

National Council Against Health Fraud
PO Box 1276
Loma Linda, CA 92354
(714) 824-4690

National Dairy Council
6300 N River Rd
Rosemont, IL 60018
(708) 696-1020

National Seafood Educators
PO Box 60006
Richmond Beach, WA 98160
(206) 546-6410

North Carolina Sea Grant
NC State University Seafood Laboratory
PO Box 1137
Morehead City, NC 28557

United States Environmental Protection Agency
(EPA)
401 M St, SW
Washington, DC 20460
(202) 382-2090

United States National Marine Fisheries Service
(NMFS)
1335 East-West Hwy
Silver Spring, MD 20910
(301) 427-2239

United States Department of Agriculture
(USDA)
14th St and Independence Ave, SW
Washington, DC 20250
(202) 447-2791

Cooperative Extension Service (CES)
Offices are located in most counties. CES
links USDA with state universities. Consult
your telephone directory.

Food Safety Inspection Service (FSIS)
USDA Meat and Poultry Hotline
14th St and Independence Ave, SW
Room 1165-South
Washington, DC 20250
(800) 535-4555

United States Food and Drug Administration
(FDA)
5600 Fishers Lane
Rockville, MD 20857
(301) 443-1544

United States Public Health Service (USPHS)
200 Independence Ave, SW
Washington, DC 20201
(301) 443-4100

119

Centers for Disease Control and Prevention
(CDC)
1600 Clifton Rd, NE
Atlanta, GA 30333
(404) 332-4597

State and County Health Departments
Offices are located in most counties. State and county health Departments are linked with the CDC, FDA, and other federal agencies. Consult your local telephone directory.

Appendix 1

Safety Recommendations for Selected Foods

Meats

Ground meats and stew meats; fresh (raw)—
beef, veal, lamb, pork

Storage—Refrigerator (40°F)—1-2 days
Freezer (0°F)—3-4 months

Cooking/comments—

• Cook all ground meats to a minimum internal temperature of 160°F, or until no longer pink and juices run clear.

• Thaw in the refrigerator (overnight for 2 pounds or less) or microwave oven (following manufacturer's instructions).

Steaks, chops, and roasts; fresh (raw)

Storage—Refrigerator (40°F)—3-5 days
   Freezer (0°F)—beef, 6-12 months; veal, 4-6
   months; lamb, 6-9 months
Cooking/comments—Cook to appropriate
   internal temperature:
   medium rare—145°F
   medium—160°F
   well done—170°F
• Thaw in the refrigerator (overnight for
   2 pounds or less) or microwave oven
   (following manufacturer's instructions).

Pork chops and roasts; fresh (raw)

Storage—Refrigerator (40°F)—3-5 days
   Freezer (0°F)—4-6 months
Cooking/comments—Cook to appropriate
   internal temperature:
   medium—160°F
   well done—170°F
• Thaw in the refrigerator (overnight for
   2 pounds or less) or microwave oven
   (following manufacturer's instructions).

Cooked meat—beef, veal, lamb, pork

Storage—Refrigerator (40°F)
   home-cooked—3-4 days
   store-cooked convenience meats—1-2 days

122

Freezer (0°F)
home-cooked—2-3 months
• Store-cooked convenience meats do not
freeze well.
Cooking/comments—Leave cooked meat at
room temperature no longer than 2 hours.
• Thaw frozen cooked meat in the refrigerator
(overnight for 2 pounds or less).
• Soups and stews will reheat more evenly
and quickly if they are thawed first.

Ham, canned (label says "Keep refrigerated")
Storage—Refrigerator (40°F)—6-9 months
Freezer (0°F)—Do not freeze.
Cooking—Fully cooked—reheat to 140°F,
if desired
Ham, fully cooked ("Smoked," "aged," or
"dried" do not mean cooked. Look for the
designation, "fully cooked." When in doubt,
cook ham as for other pork.)
Storage—Refrigerator (40°F)
whole—7 days
half—3-5 days
slices—3-4 days
Freezer (0°F)—1-2 months

Cooking/comments—Fully cooked—reheat
to 140°F, if desired
• Thaw in the refrigerator (overnight for
2 pounds or less).

Ham, dry-cured, country-style

Storage—Pantry—1 year (unopened)
Refrigerator (40°F)—2-3 months
unsoaked or cooked—2-3 months
soaked or cooked—5 days
Freezer (0°F)—Do not freeze.

Corned beef, in pouch with pickling juices
Storage—Refrigerator (40°F)—5-7 days
Freezer (0°F)—1 month (drained and
wrapped)
Cooking/comments—Cook to an internal temperature of 170°F. (Typically corned beef's
long, slow, moist cooking results in an internal temperature higher than 170°F.)
• Thaw in the refrigerator (overnight for
2 pounds or less).

Packaged luncheon meats

Storage—Refrigerator (40°F)
    opened—3-5 days
    unopened—2 weeks
Cooking/comments—Leave at room temperature no longer than 2 hours.

Hotdogs

Storage—Refrigerator (40°F)
    opened—1 week
    unopened—2 weeks
    Freezer (0°F)—1-2 months (in freezer wrap)
Cooking/comments—Leave at room temperature no longer than 2 hours.
  • Thaw in the refrigerator (overnight for 2 pounds or less).
  • Cook to 140°F or until steaming.

Chicken salad (or other store-prepared or home-prepared salad)

Storage—Refrigerator (40°F)—3-5 days
    Freezer (0°F)—These foods do not freeze well.
Cooking/comments—Leave at room temperature no longer than 2 hours, including preparation time.

Liver and other variety meats

Storage—Refrigerator (40°F)—1-2 days
   Freezer (0°F)—3-4 months
Cooking/comments—Thaw in the refrigerator
   (overnight for 2 pounds or less) or
   microwave oven (following manufacturer's
   instructions).

Pre-stuffed chops or chicken breasts

Storage—Refrigerator (40°F)—1 day
   Freezer (0°F)—These products do not
   freeze well.
Cooking/comments—Cook until the stuffing
   reaches an internal temperature of 165°F.

Bacon

Storage—Refrigerator (40°F)—7 days
   Freezer (0°F)—1 month
Cooking/comments—Thaw in the refrigerator
   (overnight for 2 pounds or less) or
   microwave oven (following manufacturer's
   instructions).

Sausage

Storage—Refrigerator (40°F)
  Raw—1-2 days
  Smoked breakfast links, patties—7 days
  Hard sausage (pepperoni, jerky)—2-3 weeks
Freezer (0°F)—1-2 months
Cooking/comments—Cook bulk (raw) and
  smoked breakfast sausage to a minimum
  internal temperature of 160°F, or until
  there is no visible pink interior.
  • Thaw in the refrigerator (overnight for
  2 pounds or less) or microwave oven
  (following manufacturer's instructions).

Meat gravy/broth

Storage—Refrigerator (40°F)—1-2 days
  Freezer (40°F)—2-3 months
Cooking/comments—Reheat until boiling, stir-
  ring frequently.

Wild game, raw

Storage—Freezer (40°F)—8-12 months
Cooking/comments—Cook to an internal temperature of 180°F.

Poultry

Chicken or turkey; fresh (raw)

Storage—Refrigerator (40°F)—1-2 days in
loose wrapping
Freezer (0°F)
whole—1 year
pieces—9 months
Cooking/comments—Ground poultry—165°F
• Whole poultry—180°F
• Breasts, roasts, thighs or wings—170°F, or
until juices run clear

Giblets (raw)

Storage—Refrigerator (40°F)—1-2 days
Freezer (0°F)—3-4 months
Cooking/comments—Cook to 170°F.

Cooked poultry

Storage—Refrigerator (40°F)
fried chicken—3-4 days
cooked mixed casseroles—3-4 days
pieces, plain—3-4 days
pieces, covered with gravy or broth—
1-2 days
nuggets or patties—1-2 days
Freezer (0°F)
fried chicken—4 months
cooked mixed casseroles—4-6 months

128

pieces, plain—4 months
pieces covered with gravy or broth—
    6 months
nuggets or patties—1-3 months

Seafood
Shrimp, fresh
Storage—Refrigerator (40°F; stored on a bed
    of crushed ice)—2 days
    Freezer (0°F)—3 months (Do not refreeze
    previously frozen shrimp.)
Cooking/comments—Buy only raw shrimp that:
- have mild odor
- have firm meat
- are not slippery
- retain their natural color

Avoid raw shrimp that:
- are bright pink or red
- have black spot

Shrimp, cooked
Storage—Refrigerator (40°F; stored on a bed
    of crushed ice)—1-2 days
    Freezer (0°F)—3 months (Do not refreeze,
    if previously frozen.)
Cooking/comments—Buy only cooked shrimp
    that have:

- red shells
- meat with a red tint
- no disagreeable odor

Avoid cooked shrimp that are displayed in contact with raw shrimp or seafood.

Clams or mussels; fresh

Storage—Refrigerator (40°F; stored in a container covered loosely with a clean, damp cloth; not in airtight containers or in water)—1-2 days
Freezer (0°F)—3 months
Cooking/comments—Buy only:
- from reputable dealers.
- live, in-shell clams or mussels with intact shells that are tightly closed or that close when handled. Soft-shell clams can't completely close their shells, but they should move when touched.

Discard any clams or mussels that are not live before cooking.

To cook (small quantities only):
- boil until shells open. Then continue to boil for 3-5 minutes.
- steam 4-9 minutes from the start of steaming.

- discard any that do not open during cooking.

Scallops, raw

Storage—Refrigerator (40°F)—1-2 days
Freezer (0°F)—3 months
Cooking/comments—Buy only scallops that:
- have a sweet odor
- are free of excess liquid

Oysters, fresh

Storage—Refrigerator (40°F; stored in a container covered loosely with a clean, damp cloth; not in airtight containers or in water)—1-2 days
Freezer (0°F)—3 months
Cooking/comments—Buy only:
- from reputable dealers.
- live, in-shell oysters with intact shells that are tightly closed or that close when handled. Discard those that die before shucking.
- shucked oysters that are plump with a natural creamy color and clear or slightly opalescent liquid. They should not contain

more than 10 percent liquid, and should have a mild odor.

To cook in-shell oysters (small quantities only):

- boil until shells open. Then continue to boil for 3-5 minutes.
- steam 4-9 minutes from the start of steaming.
- discard any clams that do not open during cooking.

To cook shucked oysters:

- boil or simmer for at least 3 minutes.
- fry in oil for at least 10 minutes at 375°F.
- bake for at least 10 minutes at 450°F.

Crabs and lobsters; whole

Cooking/comments—Buy whole crabs and lobsters live. They should show some leg movement. Lobster tails should curl under their bodies and not hang down when they are picked up.

- Discard any that die before cooking.
- Cook before refrigerating or freezing.

Crabs and lobsters; cooked

Storage—Refrigerator (40°F)—1-2 days
   Freezer (0°F)—3 months
Cooking/comments—Buy only cooked crabs
   and lobsters that:
   • have a bright red color
   • no disagreeable odor

Fish, fresh

Storage—Refrigerator (40°F)
   whole fish—in a container of crushed ice
      on the lowest shelf of the refrigerator—
      1-2 days
   fillets or steaks—waterproof containers
      buried in crushed ice on the lowest
      shelf of the refrigerator—1-2 days
Freezer (0°F)
   lean fish—6 months
   fatty fish—3 months
Cooking/comments—Buy only whole fish
   that have:
   • bright, clean, full, protruding eyes
   • bright red or pink gills that are slime-free
   • firm, elastic flesh that is not separating
   from the bone
   • shiny skin with scales that adhere tightly
   • characteristic colors and markings

133

- an intestinal cavity that is pink with a bright red blood streak
- fresh, mild (not "fishy") odor

Buy only fish steaks and fillets that:
- are moist
- have no drying or browning around the edges
- have a fresh, milk (not "fishy" odor)

Cook fish:
- to an internal temperature of 145°F for at least 1 minute
- for 10 minutes per inch of thickness at a temperature of (425-450°F). Add 5 minutes to the total cooking time if the fish is wrapped in foil or cooked in a sauce. Cook 20 minutes per inch for frozen fish. If a fish fillet is not of uniform thickness, fold the thinner part under the rest.

Seafood, commercially frozen

Storage—Freezer (0°F)—6 months

Cooking/comments—Look for frozen seafood that:
- is solidly frozen
- has no discoloration (freezer burn)
- has no objectionable odor
- is wrapped in freezer wrap that fits closely

and is undamaged
- is in uniform pieces that are not frozen together
- has intact breading or coating

Smoked, pickled, vacuum-packed and modified-atmosphere-packed seafood products

Storage—Refrigerator (40°F)—see labels for handling instructions
Freezer (0°F)—Do not freeze.

Eggs, fresh

Storage—Refrigerator (40°F)
   fresh, in shell—3 weeks
   raw yolks, whites—2-4 days
   hard-cooked—1 week
Freezer (0°F)
   fresh, in shell—Don't freeze.
   raw yolks, whites—2-4 days
   hard-cooked—don't freeze well
Use clean eggs, free of cracks.

Cooking/comments—To safely prepare basic egg dishes other than hard-cooked, cook eggs until the whites are completely coagulated and the yolks begin to thicken. They should no longer be runny, but they do not have to be hard. Once cooked, they should be served promptly.

135

• Avoid keeping broken-out eggs or prepared egg dishes out of refrigeration for
more than 1 hour, including time for
preparing and serving (but not cooking).
• Thaw frozen eggs and egg products in
the refrigerator.

Pasteurized eggs/egg substitutes
Storage—Refrigerator (40°F)
    opened—3 days
    unopened (previously frozen)—10 days
  Freezer (0°F)
    opened—Don't freeze.
    unopened (frozen)—1 year
  Thaw in the refrigerator.

Dairy Products
Milk
Storage—Refrigerator (40°F)—5 days
  Freezer (0°F)—1 month

Cheeses, hard (Swiss, brick, Cheddar, processed, etc.)
Storage—Refrigerator (40°F)—3-4 weeks
  Freezer (0°F)—These products do not
    freeze well.

Yogurt

Storage—Refrigerator (40°F)—10 days after "sell date" if unopened

Miscellaneous Foods

Mayonnaise, commercial

Storage—Refrigerate after opening (40°F)—2 months
Freezer (0°F)—Don't freeze.

Frozen dinners and casseroles

Storage—Freezer (0°F)—3-4 months. Keep frozen until ready to heat and serve.

Home-canned Foods

Home-canned meats, soups, stews

Storage—Store unopened canned meats, soups, and stews in a cool, dry place. Although canned foods lose flavor and nutrients with long storage, they remain safe to eat if the can is not bulging and its seal is not broken.
• Store opened canned food in the refrigerator (covered).
Cooking/comments—Boil all home-canned meats, soups, and stews for 15 minutes (covered).

Safe Food for You and Your Family

Appendix 2

Characteristics of Selected Contaminants

Bacteria

Bacillus cereus

Symptoms—nausea, vomiting, watery diarrhea, abdominal cramps

Associated foods—rice dishes and pasta; meat products, soups, puddings, sauces

Prevention—hold at cooked foods at 140°F or greater, cool rapidly

Campylobacter spp

Symptoms—diarrhea (sometimes bloody), fever, headache, nausea, abdominal pain

Complications—arthritis, carditis, cholecystitis, colitis, endocarditis, erythema nodosum, Guillain-Barre syndrome, hemolytic uremia

139

syndrome, meningitis, pancreatitis, septicemia

Associated foods—poultry, unpasteurized milk,
raw vegetables

Prevention—thorough cooking, pasteurization
of milk, washing raw produce

Clostridium botulinum

Symptoms—fatigue, weakness, double vision,
vertigo followed by severe nervous system
damage, respiratory paralysis; death, if not
properly treated

Associated foods—home-canned foods, smoked
and salted fish, cooked root vegetables held
at warm temperatures too long, home-
prepared garlic- and herb-flavored oils

Prevention—appropriate heat treatments,
acidulation, refrigeration

Clostridium perfringens

Symptoms—intense abdominal cramps,
diarrhea

Associated foods—meats, soups, gravies, stews,
casseroles

Prevention—hold at 140°F or greater, cool
rapidly, reheat to 165°F

140

Escherichia coli O157:H7

Symptoms—severe cramping, bloody diarrhea
Complications—hemolytic uremia syndrome, erythema nodosum, seronegative arthropathy, thrombotic thrombocytopenic purpura
Associated foods—raw or undercooked ground beef, unpasteurized milk
Prevention—thorough cooking to 160°F, pasteurization

Listeria monocytogenes

Symptoms—flu-like symptoms, septicemia, meningitis, spontaneous abortion, perinatal septicemia
Associated foods—unpasteurized milk, soft cheese, raw produce, deli items
Prevention—sanitation, thorough cooking and reheating to 165°F, pasteurization

Salmonella spp

Symptoms—abdominal cramps, diarrhea, fever, chills, headache
Complications—aortitis, cholecystitis, colitis, endocarditis, epididymoorchitis, meningitis, myocarditis, osteomyelitis, pancreatitis, Reiter's disease, rheumatoid syndromes, septicemia, splenic abscesses, thyroiditis,

141

septic arthritis (persons with sickle-cell
anemia)

Associated foods—eggs, poultry products,
meat, fish, shellfish

Prevention—thorough cooking, cleanliness and
sanitation, pasteurization, personal hygiene

Shigella spp

Symptoms—abdominal cramps, diarrhea
(stools may contain blood or mucus), fever,
vomiting

Complications—erythema nodosum, hemolytic uremia syndrome, peripheral neuropathy,
pneumonia, Reiter's disease, septicemia,
splenic abscesses, synovitis

Associated foods—salads, raw vegetables,
poultry

Prevention—personal hygiene, sewage control,
thorough cooking

Staphylococcus aureus

Symptoms—nausea, vomiting, abdominal
cramping

Associated foods—salads with protein-
containing ingredients; meat, poultry,
milk and egg products

Prevention—thorough cooking, refrigeration

Vibrio cholera
Symptoms—diarrhea (profuse, watery),
  variable fever
Associated foods—seafood
Prevention—sewage control, thorough
  cooking

Vibrio parahaemolyticus
Symptoms—diarrhea (explosive, watery),
  abdominal cramps, vomiting, headache,
  fever
Complications—septicemia
Associated foods—raw or undercooked
  shellfish
Prevention—thorough cooking, refrigeration

Vibrio vulnificus
Symptoms—chills, fever, prostration, often
  death
Associated—raw or undercooked clams and
  oysters
Prevention—thorough cooking

Yersinia enterocolitica
Symptoms—severe abdominal pain mimicking
  appendicitis, fever, diarrhea, vomiting
Complications—arthritis, cholangitis, erythema
  nodosum, liver and splenic abscesses, lym-

phadenitis, pneumonia, pyomyositis,
Reiter's disease, septicemia, spondylitis,
Stills's disease
Associated foods—chocolate milk, reconstitut-
ed dry milk, tofu, pork chitterlings, meat
Prevention—cleanliness and sanitation, person-
al hygiene, thorough cooking

Parasites

Cryptosporidium parvum

Symptoms—severe diarrhea, sometimes fever,
nausea and vomiting
Associated foods—mishandled foods, contaminated surface water
Prevention—sanitation, thorough cooking

Giardia lamblia

Symptoms—severe diarrhea
Complications—cholangitis, dystrophy, joint
symptoms, lymphoidal hyperplasia
mishandled foods
Prevention—cleanliness and sanitation, thorough cooking

Trichinella spiralis

Symptoms—muscle pain, fever

Complications—cardiac dysfunction, neurologic sequelae

Associated foods—raw or under-cooked pork or meat of carnivorous animals (bears, etc.)

Prevention—thorough cooking, freezing pork at 5°F for 30 days, irradiation

Viruses

Hepatitis A virus

Symptoms—fever and nausea; can be followed by acute hepatitis

Associated foods—raw or undercooked shellfish, mishandled foods

Prevention—thorough cooking, cleanliness and sanitation

Safe Food for You and Your Family

Index

additives, 10-11, 102-104
arthritis, 2

baby foods, 60-61
backpacking, 78-79
bacon, 126
bacteria, 11-21, 45, 139-144
barbecues, 75-77
beans, dried, 17
beef, 22, 77, 121-123
biotechnology, 110-114
birth defects, 2
bST-milk, 111-112
buffets, 28
butter, 45
buttermilk, 17

camping, 78-79
cancer, 6
canned foods,
      commercial, 31, 37, 48
   home, 20, 26-27, 97, 137
casseroles, 22, 87
catering, 94
cheese, 40, 136
chemicals, 10
chicken salad, 125
chicken, 126
childcare centers, 97-100
clams, 81, 83, 130
cleaning equipment, 45-47
contaminants, 9-12

contamination, cross, 13, 48

convenience foods, 7

cooking techniques, 49-57

corned beef, 124

crab, 82, 132-133

cutting boards, 45, 56-57

dairy products, 136-137

dating, food, 38

defects, birth, 2

donated food, 93

dry ice, 42

education, food safety, 8-9

eggs, 17, 38, 135-136

fish, 17, 77, 79-85, 133-135

Flavr Savr tomato, 111-112

foodborne illness, 2, 6-7, 9-16

frozen food, 26, 28, 38-39, 43-44, 50-51

fruit, 18-19, 44

genetically engineered foods, 110-114

gifts, food, 95-97

gravy, 127

grilling, 75-77

ham, 123-124

holiday meals, 85-91

home-canned foods, 20, 26-27, 97, 137

hotdogs, 125

ice cream, 25, 43

ice, dry, 42

illness, foodborne, 1-2, 6-7, 9-16

infants, 6

insulated coolers, 72-74

irradiation, 106-109

jelly, 40

knives, cleaning, 45

kosher food, 26

labels, food, 35-36,
    113-114
leftovers, 59-64
liver, 126
lobster, 82-83, 132-133
lunch, 64, 70, 95
luncheon meats, 125
luncheons, 93

mail-order foods, 95-97
margarine, 45
marinade, 13, 51-52
mayonnaise, 20, 137
meals, packing, 69-75
meat,
    canned, 17
    deli, 70
    raw, 64-67, 76,
    121-129
meringue, 87
microorganisms, 9-12
microwave cooking, 22,
    52-55
milk, 64, 111-112, 136
mold, 16, 40, 44
mousse, 87
mushrooms, 29

mussels, 130

nitrites, 104
nuts, dried, 17

oils, flavored, 19-20
oysters, 81, 83, 131-
    132

packaging, 7-8, 27, 31
pantry, 36, 40
parasites, 16
pasta, 18
pasteurization, 20-21
pesticides, 10, 104-105
pests, 14, 29
pets, 14
picnics, 71-75
pork, 77, 122-123
potluck meals, 91-95
poultry, 17, 22, 64-67,
    77, 128-129
power outages, 40-42
pregnancy, 6
prepared foods, 7-8
preparing foods, 47-49

preservation methods, food, 101-109

recipes, 49
refrigerated foods, 7-8, 37-38, 40, 44-45, 73
regulations, food safety, 1-2, 5
resources, 115-120
rhubarb, 9

salad bars, 28
sanitizing solutions, 46-47
sausage, 127
scallops, 81, 131
seafood, 79-85, 129-135
serving foods, 57-59
shelf life, 36
shopping for food, 25-32
shrimp, 81, 129-130
slow cooking, 55-57
smoking foods, 76-77

soft drinks, 33
soup, 98
spoiled food, 18
steak, 122
steroid medications, 6
storing foods, 35-46
street vendors, 32-33
stuffing, turkey and, 89-91
sulfites, 103-104
superchilling, 83-85

take-out food, 30
temperature recommendations, food and, 49
thawing foods, 65, 80
thermometer, usage of, 21-22
thermos, usage of, 70-71
time, contamination and, 15-16
transporting foods, 32-35
traveling, 34

turkey, 22, 89-91

United States
    Department of
    Agriculture, 5
utensils, 58

vegetables, 19, 44
viruses, 16, 144

water, purifying, 78

yogurt, 17, 137

www.ingramcontent.com/pod-product-compliance
Lightning Source LLC
Chambersburg PA
CBHW030017290326
41934CB00005B/377